A HAND BOOK
OF
AYURVEDA

VAIDYA BHAGWAN DASH

ACARYA MANFRED M. JUNIUS

CONCEPT PUBLISHING COMPANY
NEW DELHI

ISBN 81-7022-082-3

First Published 1983
Reprinted 1987, 1997, 2003

Published and Printed by
Ashok Kumar Mittal
Concept Publishing Company
A/15-16, Commercial Block, Mohan Garden,
NEW DELHI-110059

Phones : 25351460, 25351794
Fax : 091-11-25357103
Email : publishing@conceptpub.com

Introductory Notes

This Hand Book on Ayurveda is intended for students and teachers as a continuously growing series of information which constitutes the guidelines of training in this science.

The course grows directly out of the experience of teaching and practice of Ayurveda.

It has been said that a good teacher should provide only as much of information to the student at a time as the latter can absorb according to his stage of development. Information on the various aspects of Ayurveda is therefore given in stages.

Since the course consists of a growing series of volumes, we shall return again and again to each important topic in subsequent volumes. Instead of dealing with topics exhaustively in one volume, thus giving the impression of high specialisation, we shall attempt to present Ayurveda from the very start as a fully integral science with many ramifications, all of which must be taken into consideration simultaneously.

In our age of over-specialisation, where "in front of every hole of the body there sits a specialist" as a great oriental physician put it during the International Congress of Traditional Asian Medicine at the Australian National University in 1979, the re-integrating message of Ayurveda, which always treats the patient as a whole, is of vital importance.

Virtually everybody can profit in one way or the other through the study of Ayurveda. As one of the great Mother-sciences it provides valuable insight to the housewife as much as to the medical practitioner, the specialist included.

The present course constitutes the basic teaching material of the Australian School of Ayurveda in Adelaide.

Simultaneously each volume is intended as a working-book. The blank spaces on every page are intended for notes by the students or teachers. These entries could be further commentaries, drawings, records of personal experience, references to other works or information, and so forth. By adding his or her personal notes to the material provided, students participate actively in completing the great mosaic of Ayurveda during their years of study, and each volume simultaneously becomes a personal document.

Besides the present volumes, students are advised to procure the following works :

1. Fundamentals of Ayurvedic Medicine, by Vaidya Bhagwan Dash. Bansal & Co., Delhi 1980. (FAM).
2. Ayurvedic Treatment for Common Diseases, by Vaidya Bhagwan Dash. Delhi Diary Publishers, 9/172, Jor Bagh Market, New Delhi 1979. (ATCD).
3. Basic Principles of Ayurveda, by Vaidya Bhagwan Dash and Vaidya Lalitesh Kashyap, Concept Publishing Co., New Delhi 1980. (BPA).
4. Materia Medica of Ayurveda, by Vaidya Bhagwan Dash and Vaidya Lalitesh Kashyap, Concept Publishing Co., New Delhi 1980. (MMA).
5. Diagnosis and Treatment of Diseases in Ayurveda, part one, by Vaidya Bhagwan Dash and Vaidya Lalitesh Kashyap. Concept Publishing Co., New Delhi 1981. (This is the first of five volumes). (DTDA).
6. Embryology and Maternity in Ayurveda, by Vaidya Bhagwan Dash, Delhi Diary Publishers, 9/172, Jor Bagh Market, New Delhi 1975. (EMA).
7. Carka Saṃhitā, Text with English Translation and Critical Exposition, by Dr. Ram Karan Sharma and Vaidya Bhagwan Dash, Vol. 1 and Vol. 2. Chowkhamba Sanskrit Series Office, Varanasi 1976/77. (CS).

Out of these the works mentioned under 1 and 2 are necessary from the very beginning, 3-7 are also recommended to be obtained as soon as possible.

Our course contains constant references to the abovementioned works.

We hope that students of Ayurveda will find this course useful.

Delhi/Adelaide,
March 1982

The Authors

Contents

CHAPTER ONE

Basic Principles

1. What is Ayurveda?

Etymologically speaking, the Sanskrit term *āyurveda* is composed of *āyus* which means "life", and **veda** which means "knowledge" or "science".

Ayurveda is thus the Science of Life, Knowledge about Life or a Sensible Way of Living based on Knowledge.

It is also a system of medicine in the sense that it systematises and applies the knowledge about health and disease, i.e. of balanced and unbalanced states of living beings, and how unbalanced states can be corrected and the restored balance maintained.

Generally we are accustomed to the term Ayurvedic Medicine and look upon Ayurveda as a therapeutical system, perhaps unaware that the original meaning of the Greek term therapy (therapeia) means "service". One aspect of service is healing. The term Phytotherapy (from phyton="plant" and therapeia="service") thus literally means "service through plants" and not merely herbal medicine. In the original sense the term had a much wider meaning. The idea of service through plants did not only imply the administration of medicinal preparations but also knowledge about proper nutrition. Let food be your medicines and medicines your food, said Hippocrates. Phytotherapy implied the concept of living in harmony with the entire plant-kingdom which provides us with oxygen, with wood for building and for making objects and materials including paper which serves for the diffusion of knowledge, with perfumes and precious essences, with fibre for making cloth and with green manure to keep our soil healthy. The beauty of plants, specially of flowers, uplifts our emotions, we recognise the masterly touch of creation in them. The planting of forests and parks for recreation and enjoyment and the loving care of plants for the welfare of all living creatures is as much part of true phytotherapy as the preparation and administration of herbal extracts, powders or pills.

In a similar way Ayurveda embraces all aspects of well-being of living creatures, physical, mental and spiritual. *Āyus* (life) is defined as a combination (togetherness) of body, sense organs, mind and soul.

According to Ayurveda health is not merely considered to be a state of freedom from ailments or disease, but rather a state of enjoying uninterrupted physical, mental and spiritual happiness and fulfilment. The concept of true balance does not only imply correct functioning of our systems and organs, psyche and spirit, but also a balanced and creative relationship with our fellow-creatures and nature as a whole; in the closer sense, between our family members and ourselves, between our friends and ourselves, our work and ourselves, our climate and the civilization we live in and ourselves, between our ideals and customs and ourselves, between truth and ourselves, between God and ourselves and so forth. We could extend this list *ad infinitum*. It is, therefore, not surprising that Ayurveda should be concerned with every possible aspect of life. As one of the great Mother-Sciences, it developed many branches, and it is not only concerned with the well-being of humans but also of animals and plants. Caraka defines Ayurveda as "science through the help of which one can obtain knowledge about the useful and harmful types of life, happy and miserable types of life, things which are useful and harmful for such types of life, the span of life and the very nature of life".

It follows naturally that Ayurveda maintains a very open attitude towards other systems of medicine. Says Caraka: "The wise considers the entire Universe as his Preceptor, it is only the unwise who finds enemies in it. One should therefore unhesitatingly accept proper advice from whichever quarter it may come—even from the enemy—and follow it".

After the firm establishment of Yoga throughout the Western world, where nowadays millions of individuals are benefitted through its practice, the study and practice of Ayurveda is to follow naturally.

In these Course Books, the first volume of which is lying before you, we shall present Ayurveda in its proper traditional framework and leave it to the individual to test the validity of these concepts through her or his practice. The results must speak for themselves.

The present series is primarily intended as information material for students of Ayurveda. It is less of a preplanned work on this magnificent science, but rather a continuously growing source of information directly growing out of teaching experience and the practice of Ayurveda. Instead of dealing with diseases, their pathogenesis and their cure at length in only one place or chapter alone, we shall return to these again and again during the course in subsequent volumes, thus adding new information each time to what we had learned previously. In this way knowledge will be gathered like single pieces of a mosaic, which will become more and more complete with each volume.

Ayurveda is an open-minded science. In this sense, like any form of true knowledge, it has no beginning and no end, and no work written on it can ever be complete. Although being extremely coherent and logical within its own realm, it is not limited to any particular fixed dogma, but rather universal and dynamic in character, like life itself. It is motivated by the sincere desire to restore and to maintain health in the above mentioned sense.

Out of the awareness of unity of all life the sincere aspirant of Ayurveda should accustom him or herself to recite every morning the following stanza:

sarve bhavantu sukhinaḥ
sarve santu nirāmayāḥ
sarve bhadrāṇi paśyantu
mā kaścit duḥkhabhāk bhavet.

May all be happy
May all be free from disabilities
May all look to the good of others
May none suffer from sorrow.

This is the motive by which all practitioners and students of Ayurveda are perpetually guided.

2. The Universal or Eternal Nature of Ayurveda.

1. Ayurveda does not belong to any particular civilisation or country, it aims at the well being of everybody.
2. Ayurveda has no beginning and no end.
3. Ayurveda does not cater to any particular religion.
4. Ayurveda does not belong to any particular period of history.

Ayurveda is eternal for the following reasons:
It has no beginning.
It deals with such things as are inherent in nature.
Such natural manifestations are eternal.
Drugs and dietary habits may vary, but their principles remain the same.
(Compare *Caraka Samhitā, Sūtra* 30:27).

Consult: FAM p. 2

3. The Unique Features of Ayurveda.

1. Treatment of the individual as a whole.
   (Symptomatic treatment is alien to this system. Mind, body and soul are treated together).
2. Medicines and drugs are relatively cheap.
3. No unpleasant side effects but side benefits.
4. Each Ayurvedic Medicine is a tonic.
   (Penicillin is not given to healthy people, but Ayurvedic Medicines cure *and* tonify).
5. Psychosomatic concept of disease.
6. Emphasis on positive health and prevention of disease.
7. Emphasis on wholesome diet and drinks.

(If a patient keeps proper diet, where is the need for medicine? If a patient does not follow proper diet where is the need for medicine?)

8. Simple methods of diagnosis.
9. Ayurveda is near to nature.
10. Ayurveda is conducive to yogic practice. Yoga and Ayurveda go hand in hand.
11. Ayurveda maintains an open and liberal attitude towards other systems of medicine.
12. Importance of individual constitution.
Disorders are always seen on the background of the individual's constitution, the ayurvedic physician views disease through the patient.

Consult : FAM p. 4.

4. The Aim of Ayurveda.

1. Preservation of health of healthy people and to help them to attain the four principal aims of life:
DHARMA (=that which carries, *i.e.*, doing the right things which are conducive to well being of the individual and his society).
ARTHA (=wealth, gathering of the means of livelihood).
KĀMA (=satisfaction of mundane desires, passion).
MOKṢA (=attainment of salvation through liberation and God consciousness).
2. Relief of the misery of suffering patients.

Consult : BPA p. 1 and p. 53.

5. *AṢṬĀṄGA*, or the Eight Specialised Branches of Ayurveda

1. *Kāya Cikitsā* (= Body treatment, or Internal Medicine).
2. *Śālākya Tantra* (=Treatment of the diseases of the Head and the Neck, *i.e.*, Eyes, Ears, Nose, Mouth, Throat, etc.).

3. *Śalya Tantra* (=General Surgery).
4. *Agada Tantra* (=Toxicology).
5. *Bhūta Vidyā* (=Psychology, Psychiatry, also treatment of demoniac seizures).
6. *Kaumāra Bhṛtya* or *Bāla Tantra* (=Pediatrics).
7. *Rasāyana* (=Science of Rejuvenation).
8. *Vājikaraṇa* (=Sexology).

Classical works on each of these branches separately have been written by saints and scholars. Unfortunately some of these works were destroyed during the Medieval Period of Indian History.

Consult : F.A.M. p. 4.; B.P.A. p. 3 Introduction and p. 55 definition.

6. The Mythological Origin of Ayurveda And Its Downward Manifestation Into Humanity

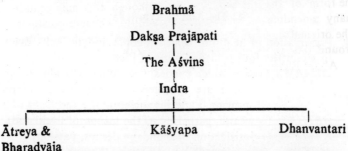

Brahmā
|
Dakṣa Prajāpati
|
The Aśvins
|
Indra
|

Ātreya & Bharadvāja	Kāśyapa	Dhanvantari
(Mainly General and Internal Medicine)	(Mainly Pediatrics)	(Mainly Surgery)

Like all Indian sciences, medicine is considered to have been originally propounded by the gods.

Brahmā, the primordial factor of the creation of the Universe, is the original propounder (not the inventor) of Ayurveda.

From Brahmā the knowledge passed to Dakṣa Prajāpati, a primordial creative sage, who is sometimes described as a son of Brahmā.

From Dakṣa Prajāpati it passed to the Aśvins. The Aśvins

became known as the divine physicians in *Svarga* or Paradise. They are also seen as the symbol of dualism acting in unison. The energies of the Moon and of Śiva are concentrated in the Aśvins. In many legends the Aśvins are associated with honey.

From the Aśvins the knowledge passed to Indra, the leader of the Gods. Indra represents the level at which energy is transmitted to the senses. Indra transmitted the knowledge to the disciples Ātreya and Bharadvāja, to Kāśyapa and to Dhanvantari.

The name Ātreya signifies the son or the disciple of Atri, a sage. Actually there were many Ātreyas, all were teachers and authors on medicine. One of them, a contemporary of the Buddha, was Professor of Medicine at the University of Taxila, where Jīvaka, Lord Buddha's physician became his disciple. Ātreya had six other famous disciples: Agniveśa, Bhela, Jatūkarṇa, Parāśara, Hārīta and Kṣārapāṇi. All of these wrote treatises on Ayurveda, most of which are lost. The work of Agniveśa, or at least a part of it, has come down to us in the form of the *Caraka Saṃhitā*, although this may contain many amendments, deletions and additions or interpolations. The original *Agniveśa Saṃhitā* may perhaps have been written around 1000 B.C. under the supervision of Ātreya.

About Bhāradvāja, the *Caraka Saṃhitā* may be quoted:

"Bhāradvāja, the ascetic of eminence, desirous of long life, having known (about Indra) approached Indra—the Lord of Immortals and protector of the devotees". (*Caraka Saṃhitā-Sūtra* 1:3).

The School of Ayurveda initiated by Ātreya and Bharadvāja specialised in Internal Medicine.

The School of Kāśyapa, another disciple of Indra, is supposed to have specialised in Paediatrics, while the School founded by Dhanvantari specialised in Surgery. Suśruta (7th c. B.C.), the famous author of the *Suśruta Saṃhitā*, an outstanding work mainly on Surgery but also including information on General Medicine, belongs to this School. Ancient Indian Surgery was extraordinarily advanced. There are descriptions of Caesarean section and of Plastic Surgery.

While the opinions as regards to the role of Brahmā, Dakṣa Prajāpati, the Aśvins and Indra are fairly consistent, there exist different views regarding the process of further downward manifestation of Ayurveda and its diffusion among humanity. We shall not enter into these controversies at this point.

Consult : FAM p. 7. BPA : Introduction p. 1.

7. A Brief Sketch of Ayurveda in History.

Vedic Period
|
Upaniṣadic Period
|
Paurāṇic Period
|
Buddhist Period
|
Post-Buddhist Period
|
Medieval Period
|
Modern Period

The Vedic Period (from ca 5000 B.C. onwards, or even earlier) is the very root of Indian Culture. The sciences of archery, fine arts, architecture and medicine are considered subsidiary subjects (*upavedas*) of the *Ṛk*, *Yajur*, *Sāman* and *Atharva Vedas*. All the Vedas contain many references to medicine, these include the *tridoṣa*-concept, the *saptadhātu*-concept, references to digestion, metabolism, anatomy and the description of diseases. Different bacteria are described as responsible for causing certain diseases. The *Ṛk-Veda* mentions 67 medicinal plants, the *Yajur-Veda* 81 medicinal plants and the *Atharva-Veda* mentions 29? medicinal plants.

The Upaniṣadic Period (from ca 1000 B.C. onwards) further systematised knowledge. The classical texts *Caraka Samhitā* and *Suśruta Saṃhitā* in their present form came down to us after the probable reactions during the 7th century B.C.. The Paurāṇic Period consolidated the knowledge further.

During the Buddhist Period (from the 6th century B.C. onwards) the Universities of Taxila (Taxashilā) and Nālanda were centres of medical science. By this time the knowledge about medicinal plants and their cataloguing had increased enormously, as a story about Jīvaka, Lord Buddha's physician, makes evident.

In order to gain admission to the Faculty of Medicine at the University of Taxila, aspiring students were put to test. They were sent to a nearby forest with the instruction to bring all those plant species not possessing medicinal properties. Most of the students returned with a number of species. Only Jīvaka returned without a single plant and told the gate keeper (Examiner) that he could not find a single non-medicinal plant. About Jīvaka many stories describing his keen sense of observation are reported.

However, surgery, which held such an important position in previous periods, underwent decline and even prohibition after the death of Lord Buddha. This was actually due to prejudice based on the following occurrence; The Buddha in his later age suffered from Fistula-in-Ano. He was operated upon and a special regimen based on Ayurvedic principles was prescribed for him after the operation. Due to the habit of taking given food, the Buddha could not observe the strict regimen given by his physicians. He is said to have eaten pork, a kind of meat strictly prohibited by his physicians, as a result of which he suffered death. This fact led to the prohibition of surgery as well as many other professions. The post-Buddhist period thus lost much of surgery, but it gained in iatro-chemistry (*Rasa Śāstra*), since medicine was forced into further research regarding other reliable healing agents. The medicinal use of mercury, gold, diamond and other metals and minerals was thus explored and systematised, and many highly complex alchemical preparations were made. Nāgārjuna, the Mahāyāna Buddhist Philosopher is supposed to have spent some of his early life in the land of the Nagas, where he learnt the secrets of the spagyric art (alchemy). He is also the author of an alchemical treatise known as *Rasa ratnākara*.

The Medieval Period was more a period of compilation than of original contribution. Many works were destroyed during this period, either by invaders or also by quarrelling Hindu and Buddhist parties, who obviously had lost the true understanding of their faith. In many ways this was a decadent period of Indian History, the consequences of which are still felt even today.

During the late 19th century and the 20th century a great revival movement of Ayurveda began. This re-established the study of Ayurveda at the Universities and led to new research and renewed interest in Ayurveda also in foreign countries.

Consult : FAM p 8-13.

8. The Philosophical Background of Ayurveda and the Concept of Creation.

Sciences in ancient India were based on various philosophical systems known as *darśanas.* These classical philosophical systems are divided into *āstika* and *nāstika darśanas.*

The *darśanas* which accept the authority of the Vedas are called *āstika,* those not based on acceptance of the authority of the Vedas are called *nāstika.*

These different philosophical systems describe truth from different points of view. Reality is not a fixed measurable entity but a variable which depends on the level and intensity of our experience. Truth has as many aspects as there are dimensions of experience. Each dimension corresponds to a particular level of reality.

Āstika Darśanas	*Nāstika Darśanas*
Sāṁkhya	*Baudha*
Yoga	*Jaina*
Nyāya	*Cārvāka*
Vaiśeṣika	
Pūrva Mimāṁsā	
Uttara Mimāṁsā or *Vedānta*	

Consult : FAM p. 15, MMA: XXXVI

According to the *Sāṁkhya* system there are 24 non living+ one living category (*Puruśa*) responsible for creation.

The system known as Yoga adds the concept of **Iśvara** (God) to these.

Vaiśeṣika accepts 9 basic categories of matter as the basis of the Universe: *pṛthvī*, *ap*, *tejas*, *vāyu*, *ākāśa*, soul, mind, time and space.

Pūrva Mimāṁsā accepts the tenets of the other *āstika* schools but holds that knowledge alone cannot give satisfaction, the soul must fulfil itself through action and religious ritual.

According to the *Uttara Mimāmsā* or *Vedānta* point of view, only *Brahman* is real and all else illusion.

Buddhist philosophy sees all reality as perpetually dynamic and denies absolutes. Therefore all forms of appearance are empty, *i.e.*, non-absolute or not possessing complete individuality.

Jaina philosophy believes in an infinite number of individual souls (monads), while the *Cārvāka* system is the materialist school of Indian Philosophy. To the open mind these systems are not necessarily contradictory to each other, since they describe reality merely from different points of view, or rather: they emphasize different aspects of reality.

Truth is relative, therefore, Indian Philosophy accepts different kinds of truth :

1. *Pāramārthika Satya* (from *paramārtha*=relating to the real), also called Eternal Truth.
2. *Vyavahārika Satya* (from *vyavahāra*=conduct, action) is truth for day to day use.
3. *Prātibhāsika Satya* (from *pratibhāsa*=appearance, illusion) is illusory truth.

Ayurveda with its open attitude, has drawn from different philosophical systems. Physical and chemical concepts and processes have been explained mainly on the basis of the *Nyāya*, *Vaiśeṣika* and also *Buddhist* philosophy, while for the explanations of the process of creation of the Universe the *Sāṁkhya*, at least in certain aspects, was considered very adequate.

According to Ayurveda the Universe evolved out of the "Unmanifested" (*Avyakta*), which implies *Prakṛti* (primordial matter) and *Puruṣa* (primordial consciousness). *Mahān* (intellect)

Creation According to Ayurveda

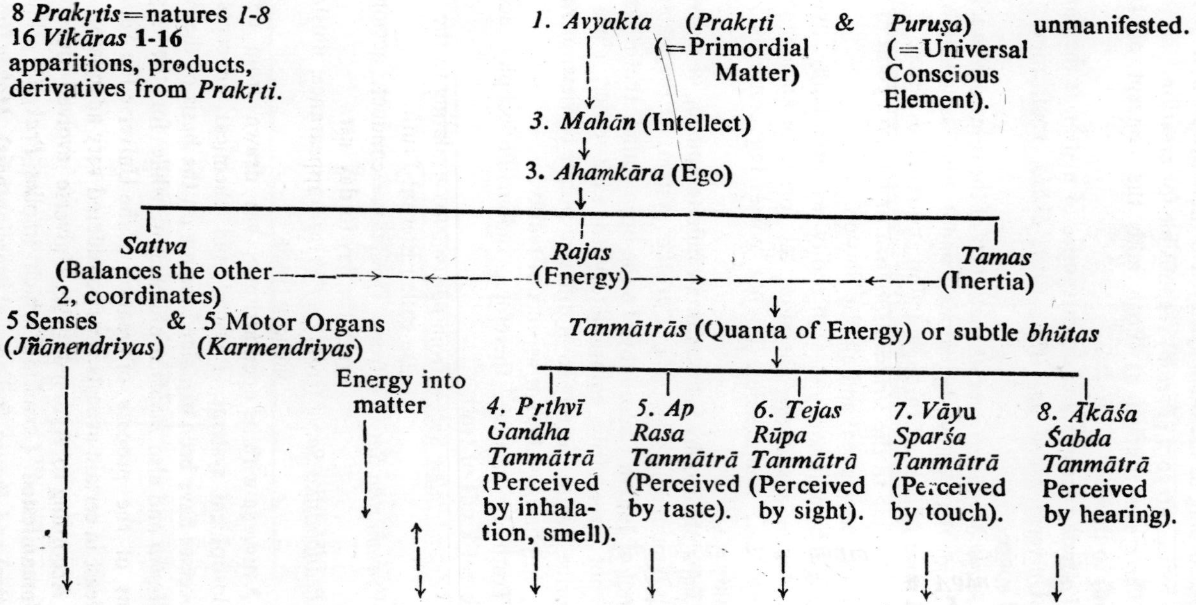
8 *Prakṛtis*=natures *1-8*
16 *Vikāras* 1-16
apparitions, products, derivatives from *Prakṛti*.
1. *Avyakta* (*Prakṛti* (=Primordial Matter) & *Puruṣa*) (=Universal Conscious Element). unmanifested.
3. *Mahān* (Intellect)
3. *Ahaṃkāra* (Ego)
Sattva (Balances the other 2, coordinates)
Rajas (Energy)
Tamas (Inertia)
5 Senses (*Jñānendriyas*) & 5 Motor Organs (*Karmendriyas*)
Energy into matter
Tanmātrās (Quanta of Energy) or subtle *bhūtas*
4. *Pṛthvī* *Gandha* *Tanmātrā* (Perceived by inhalation, smell).
5. *Ap* *Rasa* *Tanmātrā* (Perceived by taste).
6. *Tejas* *Rūpa* *Tanmātrā* (Perceived by sight).
7. *Vāyu* *Sparśa* *Tanmātrā* (Perceived by touch).
8. *Ākāśa* *Śabda* *Tanmātrā* Perceived by hearing).

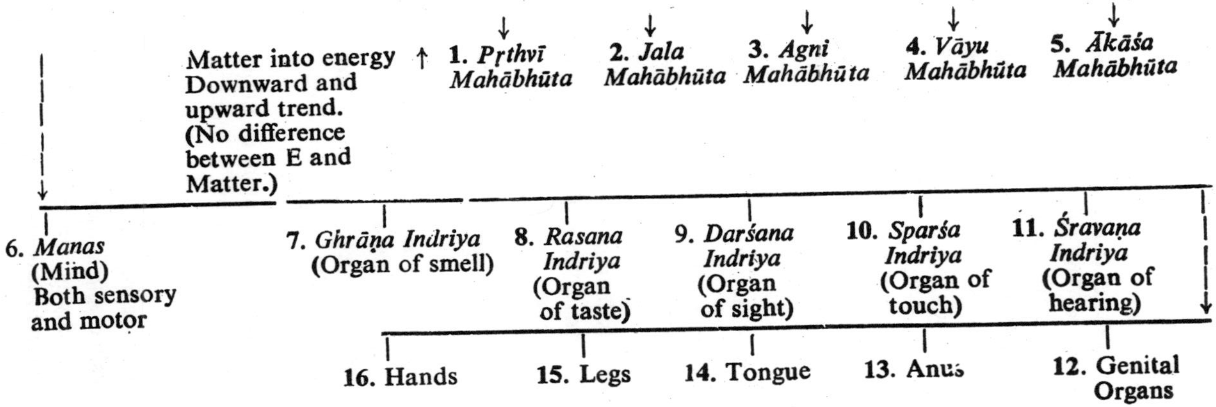

Gross elements have to be fed by *Mahābhūtas*.

Consult : **FAM p. 15 MMA p. xxxvl**

then evolves from *Avyakta*, and *Ahaṃkāra* (ego) follows. Ego has three different qualities (*guṇas*): *sattva* (the pure), *rajas* (the dynamic) and *tamas* (the inert). *Sattva* and *Rajas* together then produce 11 *indriyas* (sense and motor organs known as *jñānanendriyas* and *karmendriyas* respectively. The *guṇas tamas* and *rajas* combine to produce 5 *tanmātrās* (energy-quanta) which in their turn produce the 5 *mahābhūtas* (elements in the ancient sense, sometimes also called proto-elements). From these *mahābhūtas* the entire material world is made up.

Living beings consist of the *mahābhūtas* as well as the *indriyas*. The table in pages 12-13, illustrates the scheme.

Consult : FAM p. 15; MMA p. xxxvi

As the table indicates, energy and matter are interchangeable. The properties of the *tanmātrās* and *mahābhūtas* are:

pṛthvī : that offering resistance, solid,
ap or *jala* : the force of cohesion, liquid,
tejas or *agni* : radiation, fire,
vāyu : movement, vibration, oscillation, gaseous,
ākāśa : ether or space (root: *Kāś*="to radiate"), that which does not provide resistance.

In which way are the *tanmātrās/mahābhūtas* present in an atom?

1. Protons, neutrons, electrons, etc. represent *pṛthvī tanmātrā* or *pṛthvī mahābhūta*, also called *gandha tanmātrā*.
2. The force of cohesion (attraction) represents *ap tanmātrā* or *mahābhūta* (or *jala mahābhūta*). This is also called *rasa tanmātrā*.
3. The moving energy, which is latent in the atom in unbroken form and becomes visible only if the atom is broken, presents *tejas tanmātrā* or *agni mahābhūta*, It is also called *rūpa tanmātrā*.
4. The movement within the atom represents *vāyu tanmātrā* or *vāyu mahābhūta*. It is also called *sparśa tanmātrā*.
5. The space in which the electrons move represents *ākāśa tanmātrā* or *ākāśa mahābhūta*, which is also known as *śabda tanmātrā*.

What happens in a nuclear explosion ?

Vāyu tanmātrā acts upon the atom, *jala mahābhūta* is taken out (the force of cohesion is broken), *tejas mahābhūta* (fire) is thus liberated.

Consult : FAM p. 17

9. Molecules, Atoms and Paramāṇus.

1. *Paramāṇus*

Paramāṇu (that which is extremely subtle) may be defined as sub-atom or particle. Each *paramāṇu* has 50% of its own *tanmātrā*+4 parts of 12.5% each of the other four *tanmātrās*.

Pṛthvī *Jala* *Tejas* *Vāyu* *Ākāśa*

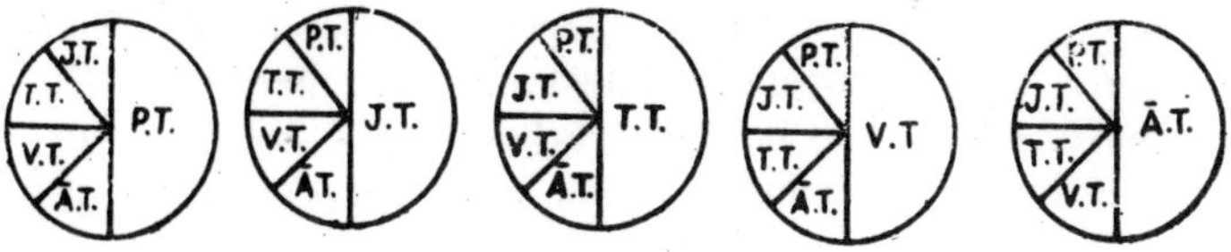

2. *Aṇu*

Each *aṇu* (the subtle or atom) consists of all five types of *paramāṇus*, which together from an *aṇu*.

Pṛthvī *Jala* *Tejas* *Vāyu* *Ākāśa*

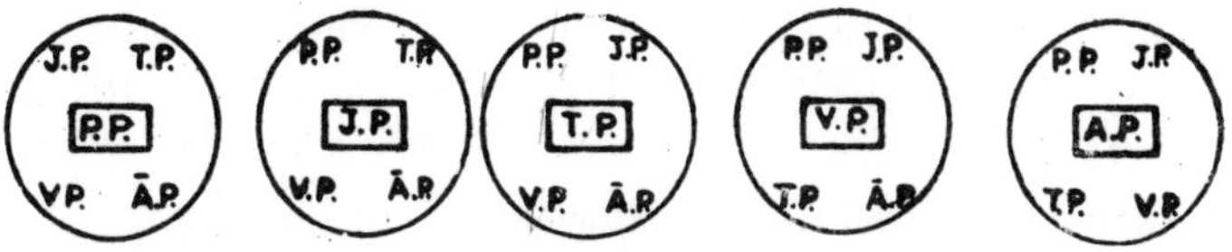

3. *Molecules*

Molecules are combinations of *anus* in different proportions, which then make water, fire, air, metals, gems, food etc.

10. The Tridoṣa Concept

According to Ayurveda, the human body is composed of three fundamental elements or categories called *doṣas, dhātus* and *malas*.

We shall deal with the subtle elements called *doṣas* first.

The *doṣas* (lit. faults) are composed of all five *mahābhūtas*, but one or the other of the *mahābhūtas* is predominant.

doṣa:	*vāyu or vāta*		*pitta*	*kapha or śleṣmā*	
predominant:	*ākāśa mahā-bhūta*	*vāyu mahā-bhūta*	*tejas or agni mahā-bhūta*	*jala mahā-bhūta*	*pṛthvī mahā-bhūta*

Correct balance between the *doṣas* is important for good health. In a balanced state the *doṣas* sustain the body. *Pitta* and *kapha* are more passive, *vāyu* is very active. The assessment of the state of balance or unbalance among the *doṣas* is very important for correct diagnosis in Ayurveda.

The three *doṣas* are:

1. *vāyu* or *vāta* (root=*vā*=*gati*-motion and *gandhana*= sensation). *Vāyu* is the originator of all movement in the body, and it governs mainly all nervous functions. There are 80 kinds of possible disturbances due to *vāyu*. Pain, stiffness, paralysis, hypertension, heart diseases—all these are caused by *vāyu*.

2. *pitta* (root *tap*=*santāpa*=heat, (also *dāha*, *aiśvarya*), governs mainly enzymes (see following pages) and hormones. *Pitta* is also responsible for digestion, pigmentation, body temperature, hunger, thirst, sight, courage etc. There are 40 kinds of possible disturbances due to *pitta*. Burning sensations, excessive body temperature, blue moles, jaundice, urticaria and pharyngitis are examples of disorders caused by *pitta*.

3. *Kapha* or *śleṣmā* (old original term used, root; *śliṣ*=*āliṅgana*=embrace or cohesion) regulates the other two. *Kapha* is responsible for the connections of joints, the solid nature of the body and its sustenance, sexual power, strength, patience etc. Among the 20 possible disturbances due to *kapha* are: anorexia nervosa, laziness, mucus expectoration, hardening of vessels, obesity, suppression of digestive power etc.

(For a more complete list of disorders caused by the *doṣas* see FAM pages 24-28).

The *doṣas* pervade the entire body, the same is true of mind. But while mind does not reach hair, nails and other waste products, the *doṣas* are present in these as well.

Each *doṣa* has three states:

1. AGGRAVATION (*vṛddhi*)
2. DIMINUITION (*kṣaya*)
3. STATE OF EQUILIBRIUM (*sāmya*).

ATTRIBUTES TO VĀYU

Attributes	*Constitutional manifestations*
1. Ununctuous (*rūkṣa*)	ununctuousness, emaciation and dwarfness of the body, longdrawn, dry, low, broken obstructed and hoarse voice; always keeping awake.
2. Light (*laghu*)	light and inconsistent gait, action, food and movement.
3. Mobile (*cara*)	unstable joints, eyes, eye brows, jaws, lips, tongue, head, shoulder, hands and legs.
4. Abundance	talkativeness, abundance in tendons and veins.
5. Swift (*śīghra cara*)	quick in initiating actions, getting irritated and the onset of morbid manifestations; quick in affliction with fear, quick in likes and dislikes; quick in understanding and forgetting things.
6. Cooling (*śīta*)	intolerance for cold things; often getting afflicted with cold, shivering and stiffness.
7. Rough (*khara*)	roughness in the hair of the head, face and other parts of the body, nails, teeth, face, hands and feet.
8. Non-slimy (*viśada*)	cracking of the limbs and organs, production of cracking sound in joints when they move.

Comp. : BPA p. 114/115, FAM p. 36.

ATTRIBUTES OF PITTA

Attributes	*Constitutional Manifestations*
1. Hot (*uṣṇa*)	intolerance for hot things, having hot face, tender and clear body, port-wine mark, freckles, black moles, excessive hunger and thirst; quick advent of wrinkles, greying of hair and baldness; presence of some soft and brown hair in the face, head and other parts of body.
2. Sharp (*tīkṣṇa*)	sharp, demonstration of physical strength, strong digestive power, intake of food and drink in large quantity, inability to face difficult situations and glutton habits.
3. Liquid (*drava*)	looseness and softness of joints and muscles; voiding of sweat, urine and feces in large quantity.
4. Fleshy smell (*visra*)	putrid smell of axilla, mouth, head and body in excess.
5. Pungent and sour taste (*kaṭu & amla*)	insufficiency of semen, sexual desire and procreation.

Comp. : BPA p. 115, FAM p. 45.

ATTRIBUTES OF KAPHA

Attributes	*Constitutional Manifestations*
1. Unctuous (*snigdha*)	unctuousness of organs.
2. Smooth (*ślakṣṇa*)	smoothness of organs.
3. Soft (*mṛdu*)	pleasing appearance, tenderness and clarity of complexion.
4. Sweet (*svādu*)	increase in quantity of semen, desire for sex-act and number of procreations.
5. Firm (*sthira*)	firmness, compactness and stability of the body.
6. Dense (*sāndra*)	plumpness and roundedness of all organs.
7. Slow (*manda*)	slow in action, intake of food and movement.

8. Stable (*sthira*)	slowness in initiating actions, getting irritated and morbid manifestations.
9. Heavy (*guru*)	non-slippery and stable gait with the entire sole of the feet pressing against the earth.
10. Cold (*śīta*)	lack of intensity in hunger, thirst, heat and perspiration.
11. Viscous	firmness and compactness in joints
12. Clear	happiness in the look and face.
	happiness and softness of complexion and voice.

By virtue of the above mentioned qualities, a man having *kapha* type of constitution is endowed with the excellence of strength, wealth, knowledge, energy, peace and longevity.

Comp. : BPA p. 115, FAM p. 44.

Although pervading the entire body, the *doṣas* are primarily prominent in certain parts of the body.

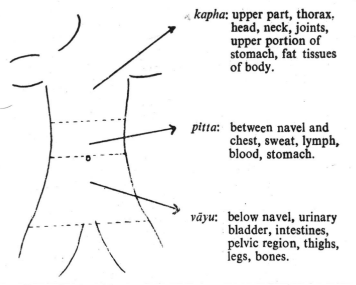

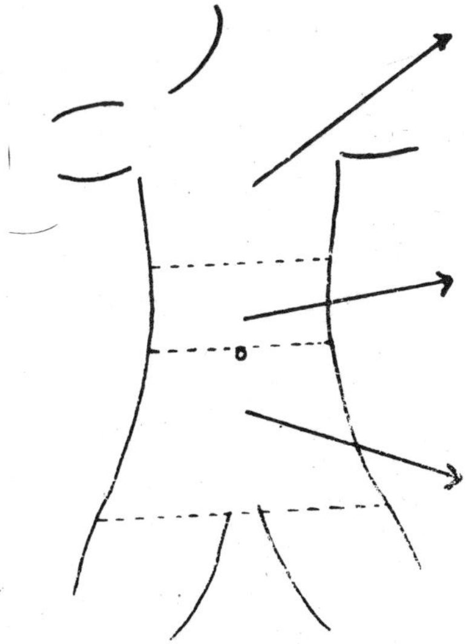

kapha: upper part, thorax, head, neck, joints, upper portion of stomach, fat tissues of body.

pitta: between navel and chest, sweat, lymph, blood, stomach.

vāyu: below navel, urinary bladder, intestines, pelvic region, thighs, legs, bones.

For a detailed list of location, function and ailments caused by the vitiation of each *doṣa* see the following pages.

Consult : FAM p. 20, 21 and 24-48.

Vāyu and its five divisions

	Location	Normal function	Ailments caused by its vitiation
1. *Prāṇa* (life breath).	Heart, also brain, face, chest, ears, nose and tongue.	Breathing and swallowing of food. "Life-giver". Sustains heart, mind, senses and intellect. Arteries veins and nerves work correctly.	Hiccup, bronchitis, āsthmā, cold, hoarseness of voice.
2. *Udāna* (rising air).	Throat, also navel, lungs, goes upward into neck and nose, downward to region of navel.	Speech and Voice. Tendency to move upward. Preservation of the body-forces, strengthens mind, memory, intellect.	Various diseases of eye, ear, nose, throat.
3. *Samāna* (one of the 5 vital airs. Lit. identical).	Stomach and small intestine. Region of navel. Moves in whole intestinal tract.	Helps in action of digestive enzymes, assimilation of end products of food and their transport into	Indigestion, diarrhoea and defective assimilation.

		various tissue elements. Digestion. Stimulates gastric juices, extracts from nourishment, those parts which are needed, transports rest to colon.	
4. *Apāna* (downward breath).	Colon and organs of Pelvis	Elimination of stool, urine, semen and menstrual blood. Keeps foetus 9 months in mother. Helps during birth. Normally presses downward.	Diseases of bladder, anus testicles, uterus and obstinate urinary diseases including diabetes.
5. *Vyāna* (that which is diffused throughout the body).	Heart	Helps in functioning of circulation channels, like blood vessels. Transports nourishing juices and blood through the body. Sweating. Opening and closing of eyelids. Yawning.	Impairment of circulation and diseases like fever and diarrhoea.

Consult : FAM p. 20; BPA p. 110,

Pitta and its five divisions

	Location	Normal function	Ailments caused by its vitiation
1. *Pācaka* (*Pācaka pitta* or *agni*. Dissolvent, digestive)	Stomach and small intestine. Duodenum	Digestion. After digestion it separates useful nourishing juices from useless ones. Supports the other 4 *pittas*.	Indigestion.
2. *Rañjaka* (is bright red, Colouring, pleasing, gratifying)	Liver, spleen and stomach	Blood formation.	Anaemia, jaundice etc.
3. *Sūdhaka* (effective, efficient).	Heart	Memory and other mental functions. The finest of all *pittas*.	Psychic disturbances.
4. *Ālocaka* (*ālocana*= seeing, consideration)	Eyes (pupils)	Vision. Helps and gives normal sight.	Impairment of vision.

5. *Bhrājaka* (that which shines).	Skin	Colour and glaze of the skin. Absorbes oily substances which are massaged into the skin.	Leucoderma and other skin diseases.

Consult : FAM p. 21.
BPA p. 111.

Kapha and its five divisions

	Location	Normal function	Ailments caused by its vitiation
1. *Kledaka* (the one who moistens)	Stomach. Is secreted in the stomach as a foamy liquid.	Moistens food which helps in digestion. Most important of the *kaphas*, nourishes the other four.	Impairment of digestion.
2. *Avalambaka* (the one who supports something)	Heart (chest)	Energy in limbs. Protects heart from excessive heat. Gives strength to heart. Acts upon heart with *rasa dhātu*.	Laziness.

3. *Bodhaka* (the one who takes care of perception)	Tongue	Perception of taste. Moistens all that touches the tongue. Tastes. When we see food we like to eat, this *kapha* forms in large quantity.	Impairment of taste.
4. *Tarpaka* (that which satisfies)	Head	Nourishment of the sense organs. Cools sense organs. Quietening effect.	Loss of memory and impairment of the functions of the sense organs.
5. *Śleṣaka* (that which connects)	Joints	Lubrication of joints. Gives solidity to joints. Through unctuousness it protects joints from heat. Makes movements smooth.	Pain in joints and impairment of the functions of the joints.

Consult : FAM p. 21, BPA p. 113.

The main locations of the doṣas in the body

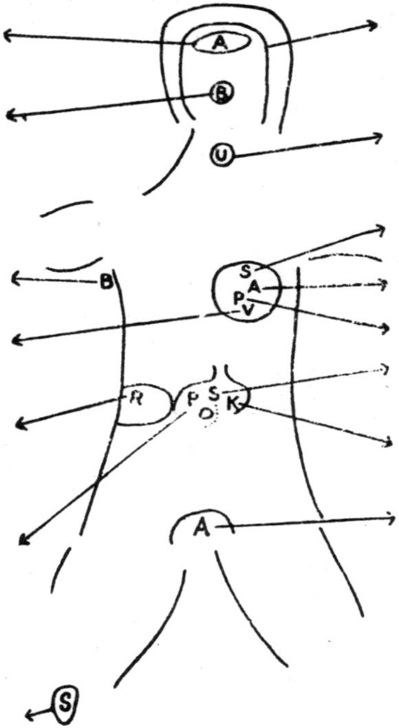
ĀLOCAKA PITTA
(in eyes)
BODHAKA KAPHA
(tongue)
BHRĀJAKA PITTA
(in skin)
VYĀNA VĀYU
(in heart, very active in skin)
RAÑJAKA PITTA (liver)
(blood formation)
PĀCAKA PITTA
(stomach, provides energy for digestion)
ŚLEṢAKA KAPHA
(joints)
TARPAKA KAPHA (head)
(nourishment of sense organs)
(*Ajñā cakra*)
UDĀNA VĀYU (throat)
(*Viśuddhi cakra*)
SĀDHAKA PITTA (in heart)
(memory, mental functions, finest pitta)
AVALAMBAKA KAPHA (heart)
PRĀṆA VĀYU (in heart)
(*Anāhata cakra*)
SAMĀNA VĀYU (stomach, intestine.) (*Maṇipura cakra*)
KLEDAKA KAPHA (stomach)
(makes sticky)
APĀNA VĀYU (bladder, prostrate, ovaries, rectum etc.) (regulates, *Mulādhāra* and *Svādhiṣhṭāna cakras*)

Consult : BPA p. 109.

11. Rasa, Vīrya and Vipāka

According to Āyurveda the essence of food does not only lie in its "combustible" or vital substances, but also in the qualities experienced by taste.

This perceivable kind of "taste essence" is called *rasa*.

Rasa is experienced through the tongue as taste as well as through the effect of the drug on the body of the consumer.

VĪRYA (potency) is registered within the body, for instance as heating, alleviating *doṣas*, stimulating digestion etc.

Two types of *vīrya* are known :

2-type vīrya, which is either

Hot (*uṣṇa*) or Cold (*śīta*), the other is the :

8-type vīrya, which is

Cold (*śīta*)
Hot (*uṣṇa*)
Unctuous (*snigdha*)
Ununctuous (*rūkṣa*)
Heavy (*guru*)
Light (*laghu*)
Dull (*manda*)
Sharp (*tīkṣṇa*).

Vīrya is an extremely active attribute of the drug.

VIPĀKA is "the taste which emerges after digestion". During digestion the ingredients of food undergo three different stages of changes because of enzyme reaction in the gastro-intestinal tract.

The product of the first stage is sweet
The product of the second stage is sour
The product of the third stage is pungent

The Table in pages 28-29 illustrates the relation between *rasa*, *mahābhūtas*, *doṣas*, metabolic effect, *vīrya* (both types) and *vipāka*.

As it can be seen, two *mahābhūtas* combine prominently to produce each of the *rasas*:

Sweet=*Pṛthvī* and *Jala*
Sour=*Jala* and *Tejas*

Saline=*Pṛthvī* and *Tejas*
Pungent=*Vāyu* and *Tejas*
Bitter=*Vāyu* and *Ākāśa*
Astringent=*Vāyu* and *Pṛthvī*.

12. The Seven Dhātus

Dhātu means: "that which enters into formation of the basic structure of the body as a whole" or which sustains the body.

The *dhātus* therefore are known as the basic tissue-elements. They have also been called the seven bodily constituents.

The seven *dhātus* are composed of all the five *mahābhūtas*, but as in case of the *doṣas* one or two *mahābhūtas* are predominant in each *dhātu*.

The *dhātus* sustain the body. The entire body is composed of the *dhātus*. (see Table in page 30 for seven *dhātus*.)

13. The Malas

Urine (*mūtra*), stool (*śakṛt*) and sweat (*sveda*) are known as the principal *malas*. They are also called "*kiṭṭa*" or waste products, (lit., "that which must go away"). There are other waste products like fatty excretions of the intestine, ear-wax (cerumen), fatty secretions of the skin, mucus of the nose, saliva, head, beard and body-hair, nails of the fingers and toes, tears etc. The *malas* are *pañcabhautika* (consisting the five *mahābhūtas*).

MALAS (Waste Products)

- Stool
- Urine
- Sweat
- Others

Stool is not only the refuse of the food taken by the individual, but it also contains substances which are eliminated from the tissue cells of the body.

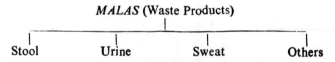

Mahābhūtas: →	Pṛthvī	Jala	Tejas	Vāyu	Akasa	
Rasa: →	Sweet	Sour	Saline	Pungent	Bitter	Astringent
Doṣas aggravated → (+ = less + + = more)	+ + *Kapha*	+ *Kapha* + *Pitta*	+ *Kapha* + *Pitta*	+ *Vāyu* + *Pitta*	+ + *Vāyu*	+ *Vāyu*
Doṣas alleviated (— less, — — more)	– – *Vāyu*	— *Vāyu*	– *Vāyu*	—— *Kapha*	— — *Kapha* — — *Pitta*	— *Kapha* — *Pitta*
Effect on Metabolism* →	+ + Anabolic	+ Anabolic	+ Anabolic + Catabolic	+ Catabolic	+ + Catabolic	+ Catabolic & Anabolic (because of association with *Pṛthvī*)

*Anabolic : building tissue, conversion of nutritive compounds into living matter.
Catabolic : breaking down tissue, breaking down compounps, often liberating energy.
Foods are dominated by *Rasa*.
Drugs are dominated by *Vīrya*.

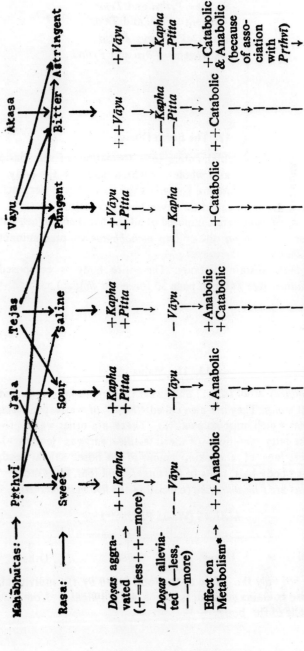

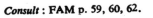

Virya (Potency 2 type) →

Virya (Potency 8 type) →

Vipaka (Taste after digestion) →

Cold → Cold Heavy ——→ Sweet

Hot → Unctuous Dull ——→ Sour

Hot → Hot Sharp ——→ Sweet

Hot → Ununctuous Light ——→ Pungent

Cold → Light ——→ Pungent

Cold → Cold Heavy ——→ Pungent

Consult : FAM p. 59, 60, 62.

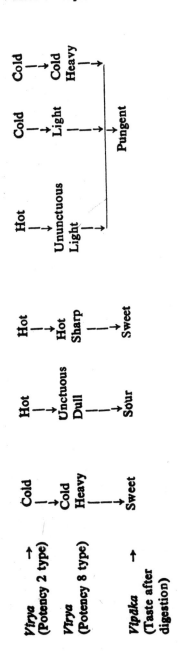

THE SEVEN DHĀTUS (Gross Tissue Elements of the Body).

Rasa	*Rakta*	*Māṁsa*	*Medas*	*Asthi*	*Majjā*	*Śukra*
(Chyle, Lymph, Plasma)	(Hemoglobin-fraction in blood)	(Muscle-tissue)	(Fat or adipose tissue)	(Bone-tissue, incl. cartilage)	(Bone-marrow)	(Semen Sperm, Ovum)
Predominant *Ap-Mahābūta*	Predominant *Tejas-Mahābhūta.*	Predominant *Pṛthvī-Mahābhūta.*		Predominant *Vāyu & Ākāśa-Mahābhūta.*	Predominant *Tejas-Mahābhūta.*	Predominant *Ap-Mahābhūta.* in finer form.

There are further *Upa-Dhātus*, which are subsidiary tissue elements, about which we shall discuss later.

Consult : FAM p. 18, BPA p. 108.

Proper digestion and evacuation of stool are of great importance for a good state of health. If there is improper evacuation, diseases do not only occur in the gastro-intestinal tract but also in other parts of the body.

Cure of rheumatism, sciatica, bronchitis and āsthmā, for instance, begins with proper evacuation of the bowels in āyurvedic treatment.

Urine, another waste product through which many body wastes are thrown out, should be passed six times per day. Adequate quantities of liquids (water) should therefore be taken.

Sweating is another way of eliminating waste products, it is common in āyurvedic treatment.

Consult : FAM p. 30, BPA p. 151.

14. The Agnis

The main task of the *agnis* (enzymes) is to help in the digestion and assimilation of food. This process takes place continuously in the body.

There are 13 groups of *agnis*:

1. One *jāṭharāgni* (*jāṭhara-agni*) which is active in the stomach and the gastro-intestinal tract. This *agni* helps to break down the food taken from outside, because food taken from outside has a different *mahābhautic* composition than our body.
2. Five *bhūtāgnis* (*pañca bhūta agnis*), mainly housed in the liver. They adapt the broken down food into a homologous chyle. This group of enzymes takes care that the *mahābhaūtic* composition of broken down food is now made into the same composition as that of the *mahābhūtas* of the body. Diet, after digestion, is thus divided into the five groups to nourish the respective attributes of the body.
3. Seven *dhātvagnis* (*dhātu-agnis*), seven groups of enzymes which synthesize the *dhātus* (tissues) out of the "cooked" food, according to requirement.

When the *agnis* work on the *dhātus*, there is formation of certain waste products. These come out in the form of excretions like ear-wax, stool (which is not only from food but also from blood, waste after enzymatic action, etc.) and discharges from the nose, eyes, etc.

We can thus see that each of the seven *dhātus* and five *mahābhūtas* has its own *agni*.

Here follows a schematic survey of the *agnis* and their activities :

I. One Jātharāgni

Saliva, hydrochloric acid, bile, pancreatic juice etc. break up food. Several enzymes break down food into molecules.

↙ ↘

Āhārarasa (Chyle) is absorbed into the body through villi and then goes to the liver — *Mala* (=Feces)

↓

Here the action of the

↓

II. Five Bhūtāgnis

begins. Chyle is made homologous, After this it circulates in the blood channels in the form of

↓

Rasa (Plasma, Lymph), which is the nutrient fluid circulating in the body, which has the material for all the seven types of *dhātus*. Now begins the work of the

↓

III. Seven Dhātvagnis

which synthesize the tissue elements. Each of these processes of synthesis also results in some waste products. The processes are as follows :

Synthesized into: ↓		*Waste Product:* ↓
	1. RASADHĀTVAGNI	
Rasa, which is acted upon by :		*Kapha* (Phlegm, not to be confused with *kapha doṣa*), this goes into feces.
	2. RAKTADHĀTVAGNI	
Hemoglobin synthesized		Bile is formed into feces.
	3. MĀṀSADHĀTVAGNI	
Muscle tissue synthesized		All excreta (eyes, ears, mouth etc.)
	4. MEDHODHĀTVAGNI.	
Fat synthesized (adipose tissue)		Sweat, which is excreted from the body. (In this way fat becomes pure).
	5. ASTHIDHĀTVAGNI	
Bone and Cartilage synthesized		Hair as a waste product. (If something is wrong with the hair therefore, we give medicines to correct *asthi*).
	6. MAJJĀDHĀTVAGNI	
Bone Marrow (white and red) synthesized		The glaze of the eyes is the waste product.
	7. ŚUKRADHĀTVAGNI	
Semen, Sperm, Ovum synthesized, + *Ozas* (Energy, glaze of the body).		Beard is the waste product with men, in females: secondary sexual characteristics.

"The excellent essence of the *dhātus* beginning from *rasa* and ending in *śukra* is called *ojas*. This *ojas* is also called *bala* in the context of the medical science. Because of strength, there is stability and nourishment of the muscle tissue and the person remains undeterred in all efforts. He gets endowed with excellence of voice and complexion. His external sense organs and internal senses are capable of performing their activities with their full abilities." (BPA p. 294)

As the bees collect honey from the essence of flowers, similarly *ojas* is collected from the essence of the tissue elements by the *agnis* like *pācaka* etc. The one which dwells in the heart and which is predominantly white and slightly reddish as well as yellowish in colour is known as *ojas* of the body. If the *ojas* is destroyed, the human being succumbs to death. (BPA p. 295)

15. Āma and its Formation

If there is a diminuition of *agni* (*agni-māndya*), i.e. when a repression of the above mentioned process takes place and in some channels correct processing does not take place, *ĀMA* is formed. Instead of moving correctly, this *āma* settles down in different parts of the body, for instance lungs, heart or any viscera. (viscus=any organ enclosed within one of the four great cavities, the cranium, thorax, abdomen or pelvis; specially an organ within the abdominal cavity). *Āma* mixed with *doṣas* goes to the site of manifestation of a disease, thus signs and symptoms become manifest, for instance bronchial āsthmā. The first question to ask in such cases is: where was the *agni* affected? In case of bronchial āsthmā: is your digestion good? Regular bowel movements?

Therefore emetic and purgative treatment would be the first step of the cure.

Āmaya means disease, diseases are invariably caused by *āma*.

Internal diseases start with *āma*.

Diseases taken from outside end with producing *āma*.

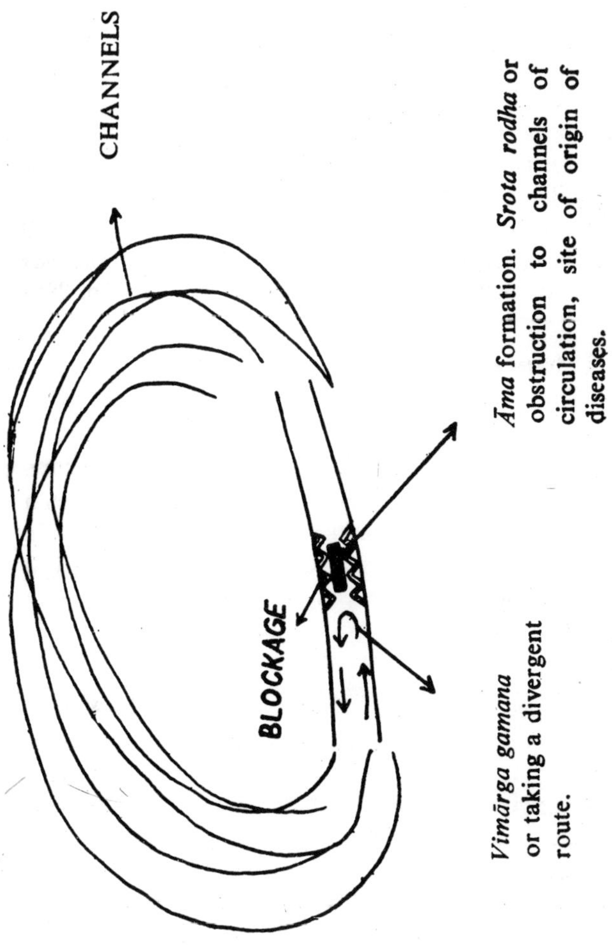
CHANNELS
BLOCKAGE
Āma formation. *Srota rodha* or obstruction to channels of circulation, site of origin of diseases.
Vimārga gamana or taking a divergent route.

Because of *āma* the *agnis* are affected, and if "uncooked" food remains, the channels get obstructed. *Āma* can get into any part of the body. Usually the organ which is stressed and thus weakened, or the organ which is similar in *mahābhautic* composition accept the *āma* more easily. If *Udāna-Vāyu* is aggravated for instance, the *āma* will go to the lungs, heart etc.

Consult : BPA p. 137 140—142.
FAM p. 105.

16. The 13 Categories of Srotas (Channels of Circulation).

The body contains a large number of channels through which the basic tissue elements, *doṣas* and waste products circulate. These channels are called *srotas* (actual plural is *srotāṁsi*).

Thus for instance, the *srotas* are responsible for carrying products of food from the gastro-intestinal tract to the basic tissue elements as nourishment.

The *srotas* include all big channels of the body like the gastro-intestinal tract, are arteries, veins, lymphatics and the genito-urinary tract, as well as very fine channels like the capillaries.

For proper functioning of a healthy body the *srotas* must remain unblocked and circulation must proceed in an uninterrupted way. If the circulation in the *srotas* is impaired or stopped, the circulating substance accumulates in the channels and metabolism of the tissues is affected. This gives rise to *āma*. *Āma* thus produced may circulate in the body through other channels which are still functioning.

Here follows a Table of the 13 groups of *srotas*, which includes their names and functions as well as possible causes and signs of their vitiation:

Name & Function	Controlling Organ	Causes of Vitiation	Signs
1. *Prāṇa vaha Srotas.* (Carrying vitality, vital breath).	Heart and Alimentary tract.	Wasting, suppression of natural urges, intake of un-unctuous food, exercise while hungry.	Long, restricted, shallow & frequent breathing. (Asthmā is connected with this).
2. *Udaka vaha Storas.* (Carrying water, fluid part of body).	Palate, Pancreas.	Exposure to heat, indigestion, excess of alcohol, intake of excessively dry food and excessive thirst.	Dryness of palate, lips, tongue and throat.
3. *Anna vaha Srotas.* (Carrying food which is taken from outside).	Stomach.	Untimely food, excessively large quantities of food, unwholesome food, less power of digestion.	Loss of appetite (Anorexia), indigestion, vomiting.
4. *Rasa vaha Srotas.* (Carrying chyle, lymph, plasma).	Heart and ten vessels connected with heart.	Worry and intake of excessively heavy, cold and ununctuous food.	Anorexia, disgeusia, ageusia, nausea, heaviness, drowsiness, fainting, anaemia, impotency.

5. *Rakta vaha Srotas.* (Carrying blood, specially hemoglobin fraction of blood).	Liver, Spleen.	Irritant, hot and unctuous food, excessive exposure to sun and fire.	Obstinate skin diseases, bleeding, abscesses, inflammation in anus and genital organs.
6. *Māṁsa vaha Srotas.* (Carrying ingredients of muscle tissue).	Tendons, Ligaments, Skin.	Sleeping immediately after meals, frequent intake of heavy and gross food.	Granuloma,[1] Myoma,[2] Piles, Uvulitis,[3] Goitre Adenitis, Tonsilitis, many cancer types as well as non-malignant growths.

1. Granuloma : swelling composed of granulation tissue.
2. Myoma : any tumor derived from muscle.
3. Uvula : the conical appendix hanging from the edge of the soft palate.

7. *Medo vaha Srotas*. (Carrying ingredients of fat tissue).	Kidneys, Omentum (fat tissue in abdomen).	Lack of exercise, day sleep (suppresses enzymes & digestion), excessively fatty food, alcohol.	Obstinate urinary disorders, including diabetes.
8. *Asthi vaha Srotas* (Carrying nutrient ingredients for bone tissue).	Hip Bone.	Excessive exercise, involving friction of bones, intake of *vātika* type of food (food producing *vāyu*).	Cracking nails & teeth, pain in bones, change in hair (because hair is excreta of *asthi*).
9. *Majjā vaha Srotas*. (Carrying nutrient ingredients of marrow).	Bones, Joints.	Contradictory (incompatible) food, injury to bone marrow by crushing, compression etc. Incompatible foods: for instance fish and milk or honey in hot drinks.	Pain in joints, giddiness, fainting, loss of memory, black-outs (entering into darkness), also deep abscesses.
10. *Śukra vaha Srotas*. (Carrying semen and ovum and nutrient ingredients for these).	Testicles, Ovary.	Sex at improper time, unnatural sex, suppression or excess of sex.	Impotency infertility, abortion, defective pregnancy.

11. *Mūtra vaha Srotas.* (Carrying urine)	Kidneys, Bladder.	Food, drinks & sex during urge for micturition, suppression of urge for micturition, specially by those suffering from wasting.	Excessive quantities or no urine. Frequency of urination, thick urine.
12. *Varco vaha* or *Purīṣa vaha Srotas* (Carrying feces)	Colon, Rectum.	Suppression of urge to pass stool. Taking of focd before digestion of previous meal. Weak power of digestion.	Less or excessive quantity of stool, hard (scybalous), stool.
13. *Sveda vaha Srotas.* (Carrying sweat).	Fat tissue, Hair-Follicles.	Excessive exercise, anger, grief, fear, exposure to heat.	Absence of or excessive perspiration. Roughness of skin. Horripilation (hair-erection). Burning sensation in skin.

Consult: FAM p. 31, 33, 34.

Prakṛti (Constitution)

When the sperm and the ovum unite in the uterus to form a zygote, the *doṣas* decide the physical constitution (*prakṛti*) of the child.

Four principal factors are responsible for the *prakṛti* of an individual:

1. The paternal factor.
2. The maternal factor.
3. The state of the womb of the mother and the season.
4. The food of the mother.

If the state of balance among the *doṣas* is very disturbed, there may be prevention of conception of growth of the zygote or malformation of the embryo.

If there is only moderate excess in one or two of the *doṣas*, this will determine the physical constitution (*prakṛti*) of the child. This constitution remains with the individual throughout each life. It does not change during the life span. In this way there are seven basic types of constitution or *prakṛti*:

1. *Vāta* or *Vāyu-Prakṛti.*
2. *Pitta-Prakṛti.*
3. *Kapha-Prakṛti.*
4. *Vāta-Pitta-Prakṛti.*
5. *Pitta-Kapha-Prakṛti.*
6. *Vāta-Kapha-Prakṛti.*
7. *Sama* (balanced) *Prakṛti.* (This is the best constitution, but it is rare).

An individual of *Vāta-Prakṛti* is more likely to get *vāta* (*vāyu*) type of diseases of a more serious nature, while those of the other two *doṣas* would be easily curable. Such an individual should avoid factors aggravating *vāyu.*

Pitta-Prakṛti individuals are more likely to get *pitta* types of diseases, and *Kapha-Prakṛti* types would have to be more careful about the *kapha* types of diseases. (For diseases caused by the *doṣas* see the detailed list in FAM p. 24-28).

For this reason medicines according to Āyurveda are always given in accordance with the patient's constitution. Quinine, for instance, can safely be given to a *Kapha-Prakṛti* person. It will be less suitable for a *Vāta-Prakṛti* person and harmful to a *Pitta-Prakṛti* person.

Consult: FAM p. 41.

17 a. Composition of the Foetus.

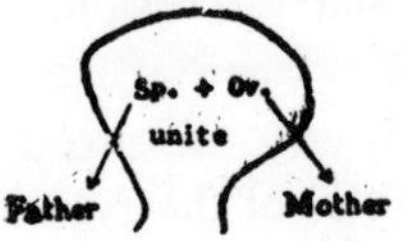

Soul (*jīvātman*) from past life enters the united stuff to animate it. This is then known as embryo (*garbha*). The soul plays the most important role by providing the vitality to the embryo.

Sperm and ovum are supplied by the father and the mother, both of these have their particular *mahābhautic* composition.

Nutrition, equally of a certain *mahābhautic* composition, is provided by the mother.

Soul (*jīvātman*), Mind (*manas*), Intellect (*buddhi*) and four of the *mahābhūtas* (*pṛthvī jala, tejas* and *vāyu*) remain suspended and then enter the cell. (Since *ākāśa-mahābhūta* is omnipresent it does not transmigrate).

The activity of the soul begins after the 4th month.

Consult: Embryology and Maternity in Āyurveda, p. 3.

17 b. Classification of Mental Faculties.

Just like there are varieties in physical constitution, there are different categories of mental faculties. These are divided into three groups according to the *guṇas* : *sāttvika, rājasika* and *tāmasika*.

Traditionally 15 types of archtypal categories are described in the texts. Of these seven are *sāttvika*, six are *rājasika* and three are *tāmasika* in character.

Here follows a survey of the categories :

Comp. : FAM p. 55-59,
BPA p. 181.

I. The seven *sāttvika* types of *prakṛti*:

1. *Brāhma* (sharing the traits of *Brahmā*)	1. Purity and love for truth. 2. Sincerity in effort. 3. Offering prayers to the gods and preceptors. 4. Respect for guests. 5. Endeavour for acquiring knowledge.
2. *Māhendra* (sharing the traits of *Mahendra*)	1. Having great fame and courage. 2. Obedience. 3. Constant devotion to scriptural studies. 4. Proper maintenance of servants.
3. *Vāruṇa* (sharing the traits of *Varuṇa*)	1. Liking for cold things. 2. Tolerability. 3. Coppery colour. 4. Greenish colour of the hair. 5. Pleasing talks.
4. *Kaubera* (sharing the traits of *Kubera*)	1. Disposition to work as a moderator. 2. Tolerability. 3. Acquiring and accumulating wealth. 4. Great power to deliver goods.
5. *Gāndharva* (sharing the traits of *Gandharva*)	1. Liking for scents and garlands. 2. Desire for dance and music. 3. Desire to move about.
6. *Yāma* (sharing the traits of *Yama*)	1. Observance of the propriety of actions. 2. Initiation of strong action. 3. Fearlessness. 4. Memory and purity. 5. Freedom from attachment, illusion, fear and jealousy.

7. *Āṣra* (sharing the traits of a *ṛṣi*)	1. Devotion to penance and sacred rituals. 2. Celibacy, oblation to fire and study. 3. Material and spiritual knowledge.

II. The six *rājasika* types of *prakṛti* :

1. *Āsura* (sharing the traits of an *asura*)	1. He is endowed with wealth. 2. Terrifying, brave, cruel and envious. 3. Liking for enjoyment alone. 4. Desire for satisfying the belly.
2. *Sārpa* (sharing the traits of a snake *sarpa*)	1. Sharpness, deceptiveness, cowardice, cruelty and intelligence.
3. *Śākuna* (sharing the traits of a bird *śakuni*)	1. Excessive indulgence in sex. 2. Frequent intake of food. 3. Anger and instability.
4. *Rākṣasa* (sharing the traits of a *rākṣasa*)	1. Onesided thinking. 2. Anger and envy. 3. Absence of religious mind. 4. Indulgence in self-praise.
5. *Paiśāca* (sharing the traits of a *piśāca*	1. Liking for taking left-out food. 2. Sharpness. 3. Liking for bravery. 4. Fondness of women. 5. Shamelessness.
6. *Praita* (sharing the traits of a *preta*)	1. Desire for not sharing enjoyments. 2. Laziness. 3. Miserable disposition. 4. Jealousy. 5. Greediness. 6. Less liking for charity.

III. The three *tāmasika* types of *prakṛti* :

1. *Pāśava* (sharing the traits of an animal *paśu*)	1. Lack of intelligence. 2. Sluggishness. 3. Indulgence in sex during dream. 4. Disobedience.

2. *Mātsya* (sharing the traits of a fish *matsya*)	1. Instability. 2. Lack of wisdom. 3. Cowardice. 4. Desire for water. 5. Mutual destruction of each other.
3. *Vānaspatya* (sharing the traits of vegetation *vanaspati*)	1. Liking to stay in only one place. 2. Liking only for taking food. 3. Absence of *sattva* (mental faculty), *dharma* (religion, sense of duty), *kāma* (desire) and *artha* (wealth).

18. The 13 Natural Manifested Urges and their Suppression (Vega-Dhārana).

(*Vega*=sudden impulse, *dhārana*=preserving, holding).

Natural Urge	*Signs of Suppression.*
1. *Micturition.* (Normal : no urine at night 6 x during the day)	Pain in bladder of genital organs, dysuria, headaches, distension in lower abdomen. Treatment : massage, tub-bath (hot), nasal drops. *Apāna-vāyu* is affected. *Vāyu* is cold.
2. *Defecation.* (Normal : 2 x per day. Take food only after complete elimination of stool and urine.)	Colic pain, headache, constipation, cramps, distension of abdomen. Treatment : Fomentation, tub-bath. Fomentations (*svedana*) are of 13 types.
3. *Seminal Ejaculation.*	Pain in genital organ, testicles, cardiac pain, retention of urine. Treatment : massage, tub-bath, enema.
4. *Flatus.*	Constipation, distension of abdomen, pain, exhaustion.

	Treatment : Fomentation, suppositories enema, carminative foods and drinks.
5. *Vomiting.* (Natural urge, not the induced type)	Itching, Urticaria, Anorexia, Oedema, Anaemia, Fever, Nausea, Erysepelas (a form of acute streptococcal cellulitis involving the skin). Treatment : Smoking, fasting, exercise, purgatives.
6. *Sneezing.*	Torticolis (stiffness of neck muscles), headache, facial paralysis, hemicrania, weakness of sense organs. (Sense organs controlled by nose). Treatment : massage, fomentations of head and neck (natural terpentine in hot water), nasal drops, butter.
7. *Eructation.* (Normally after taking areated water)	Hiccup, Dispnoea, Anorexia, Tremor, Malfunctioning of heart and lungs. Treatment : Carminatives, Purgation. *Sukumāra Ghṛta* : is an āyurvedic preparation from castor oil+butter+the root of a drug called *Puṇarnavā* (a root which rejuvenates the body, which is also used in early stages of cataract). *Sukumāra Ghṛta* is also used in cases of infertility in ladies.
8. *Yawning.*	Convulsions, Numbness, Tremor. Treatment : Drugs for alleviation of *vāyu*.

9. *Hunger.*	Emaciation, weakness, malaise, anorexia, giddines. Treatment : Unctuous, hot and light food.
10. *Thirst.* (1/4 of the stomach should be filled with liquid. Bulky persons : take drinks before food, (this reduces appetite). Lean and thin persons : drink after food. Normal persons : drink during food.	Dryness of throat and mouth, deafness, exhaustion, cardiac pain. Treatment : cold and refreshing drinks.
11. *Tears* (Weeping).	Rhinitis, eye diseases, heart diseases, anorexia, giddiness. Treatment : Sleep, wine, consolation.
12. *Sleep.*	Yawning, malaise, drowsiness, headache, heaviness in eyes. Treatment : sleep, massage of the body.
13. *Breathing.*	Phantom tumors, heart disease, fainting. Treatment : alleviation of *vāta* through drugs.

All urges are regulated by *vāyu*: *apāna* is responsible for elimination, *samāna* for digestion.

Prāṇa and *apāna* are closely connected (sympathetic and parasympathetic nervous system).

The six *cakras* control *prāṇa* and *apāna*.

Mulādhāra and *Svādiṣṭhāna*=*apāna*.

Anāhata=*prāṇa*.

Viśuddha=*udāna*.

The mind is controlled by *prāṇa vāyu*.

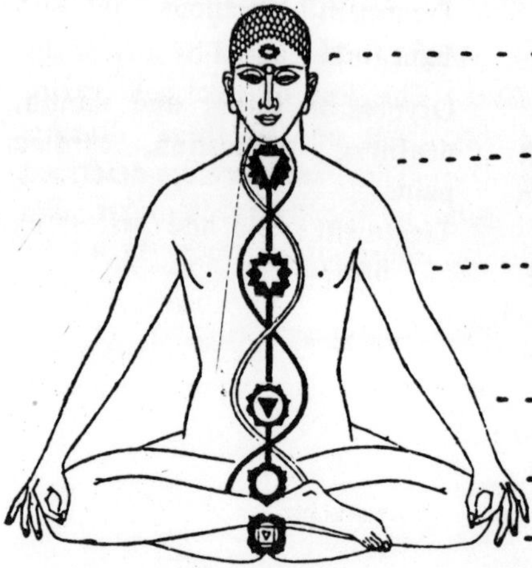

Consult : BPA p. 95.
FAM p. 149.

19. The Classification of Diseases

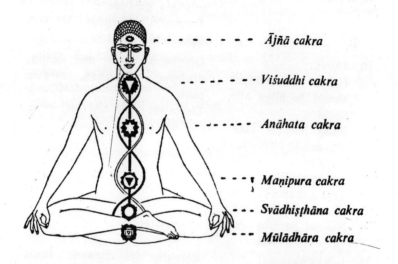

On the basis of the causes of their origin, diseases are classified into three main categories:

1. *Ādhyātmika*=diseases taking origin from factors within the body of the individual, including psychosomatic diseases.
2. *Ādhibhautika*=diseases caused by external physical factors like germs, accidents etc.
3. *Ādhidaivika*=diseases taking origin from providential causes, planetary influences, seasons etc.

There are three further sub-classifications of *ādhyātmika* diseases:

a. *ādibalaja*=hereditary diseases.
b. *janmaja*=congenital diseases.
c. *doṣaja*=caused by *doṣa* aggravation.

Diseases are further classified into two broad categories:

I. *Nānātmaja*=diseases invariably caused by a particular *doṣa*. (For instance paralysis, which involves only *vāyu*). sec FAM p. 24.

II. *Sāmānyaja*=diseases which can be caused by any of the three *doṣas*. The line of treatment varies considerably from one of these diseases to the other. They are therefore described in great detail in the āyurvedic texts. We shall discuss more about these at a later stage.

20. Disease Manifestation

Causative Factors.

Food, drink, regimen, seasonal effects, mental stress etc. leads to:

Suppression of enzyme activities. This leads to:

Āma-Formation (Uncooked material), which.

Site of origin of a disease.	→ *Obstructs the channels of circulation*, therefore there is need of a: ↓
Path of transportation.	→ *Divergent path*, and finally the result is: ↓
Site of manifestation.	→ *Affliction of a viscera.*

21. Names of Diseases

Āyurvedic texts are written in Saṁskṛt. Diseases have been named on the basis of either of the following categories.

1. *Indication of miseries.* The name often means pain or distress. *Jvara* (fever), for instance implies a painful condition. *Jvara* actually means pain.
2. *Indication of important symptoms.* For instance *atisāra* (diarrhoea). The term *ati saraṇa* implies frequent loose motions.
3. *Indication of important signs.* For instance *pāṇḍu* (anaemia), because of the yellowish pallor (*pāṇḍutā*) associated with the disease.
4. *Indication of the principal nature or character of the disease.* For instance *arśas* (piles), "that which gives miseries like a constant enemy".
5. *Indication of the important doṣa involved.* For instance the term "*vāta-roga*" is used for nervous disorders because of the invariable association of *vāyu* in such conditions.
6. *Indication of the principal organ affected.* For example *grahaṇī* (sprue-syndrome), because of the affliction of *grahaṇī* (small intestine, specially the duodenum).

CHAPTER TWO

The Practice of Medicine

1. The Examination of Patients (Rogī-Parīkṣā)
General Considerations

Consult : FAM p. 93, BPA p. 87, DTDA p. X.

For the examination of any Phenomena in the Universe in general and the patient in particular, the following three methods are prescribed:

1. *Pratyakṣa* (Direct observation)

   This is done through the senses: seeing, hearing, smelling, touching, (tasting). A direct contact between the senses and the object of the senses is established.

2. *Anumāna* (Inference)

   When there is excessive dense smoke coming out of the windows of a house, the deduction is that fire is in that house. Similarly the observation of certain substances under a microscope (for instance stool or sputum) may allow for certain deductions regarding the state of health of a person. Inference is very important in medical practice.

3. *Śabda* (Authoritative statement)

   Enlightened and experienced experts have left a treasure of authoritative statements regarding diseases. Equally the patient has to be interrogated closely to determine the exact nature of a disease. Eventually the patient's relatives have to be interrogated as well. In this way previously experienced diseases, recurrences etc. are recorded.

A brief examination of a patient procedes in three steps:

1. *Darśana* (Visual observation)
2. *Sparśana* (Touch)
3. *Praśna* (Interrogation)

For a more detailed examination the following eightfold method is prescribed:

1. *Nāḍī-Parīkṣā* (Pulse examination)
2. *Mūtra Parīkṣā* (Urine examination)

   With these two we shall deal in more detail on the following pages.

3. *Mala-Parīkṣā* (Stool examination)

   For instance if stool sinks in water, there is much *āma* in the body, if it floats on water, there is no *āma* in the body.

4. *Examination of Eyes*

   Those of a person suffering from *vāyu* diseases will be dry and smoky and the patient will complain of burning eyes. Yellowish tinge in the white of the eyes, aversion to light + burning sensation indicate *pitta* type of diseases. Unctuous and dull eyes indicate *kupha* predominance.

5. *Examination of the Tongue*

   When the tongue is cold, rough and cracked, *vāyu* is aggravated.
   A red or blue tongue indicates *pitta* aggravation.
   A white and slimy tongue indicates *kapha* aggravation.
   If the tongue is black and there are thorny eruptions, all the *doṣas* are aggravated.

6. *Examination of the Skin*

   Skin hot to the touch indicates *pitta* aggravation.
   Cold skin indicates *vāyu* aggravation.
   Moist or wet skin indicates *kapha* aggravation.

7. *Examination of Nails*

   For instance cracked and dry nails indicate *vāyu*.
   Red or yellowish nails indicate *pitta*.

8. *Examination of Physical Features*

   Vāyu dominated patients usually have dry and cracked skin and hair. They do not like cold things and tend to be impatient, lacking in memory and intellect, but tend to be talkative.

Pitta dominated patients are frequently thirsty and hungry. Their skin is hot to the touch and often yellowish. Their palms of the hands, soles of the feet and face are frequently of coppery colour. They tend to be egocentric and aggressive and have less hair. Frequently their hair has a reddish tinge. *Kapha* dominated patients have compact joints, bones and muscles, there is no excess of thirst, hunger, grief and pain.

The following aspects of patients need to be taken closely into consideration:

(a) *Prakṛti* (Physical and psychic constitution)

(b) *Vikṛti* (Nature of the disease of the patient)

(c) *Sāra* (Excellence of the tissue elements of the patient)

(d) *Saṁhati* or *saṁhanana* (Compactness of the patient)

(e) *Pramāṇa* (Measurement of the patient)

(f) *Sattva* (The will power of the patient)

(g) *Sātmya* (The wholesomeness of the patient, for instance whether he is a drinker, vegetarian etc.

(h) *Vayaḥ* (The age of the patient)

According to Āyurveda man should live 108 years. Age is divided into 10 stages, diseases during each of these stage s need different treatment. For instance, till the age of 10, *kapha* is aggravated, from 10 to 20 years, the age of youth, *pitta* is aggravated. From 30 to 40 wisdom is gathered, from 40 to 50 metabolic changes take place and in old age *vāyu* tends to be aggravated.

2. Pulse-Examination (Nāḍī-Parīkṣā)

Consult : BPA Introd. p 37, 489. FAM p. 93.

Pulse examination is carried out with the help of the radial artery. The index, middle and ring-fingers of the right hand are used in pulse examination.

The index finger is placed about the width of the index of the patient below the root of the thumb, the other two fingers are placed next to the index.

The following rules have to be observed in pulse examination:

1. Examination is perferably carried out early in the morning after ablutions, when the patient's stomach is empty. Don't examine the pulse immediately after bath or oil massage, nor when the patient is hungry or thirsty. Examination can also be carried out in the afternoon, but the patient must not have taken food for three hours.
2. The right pulse of men and the left pulse of women are examined.
3. The mind of the examiner has to be in a state of concentration.
4. The examination of the pulse is repeated at least three times. Each time the pulse is gently and evenly pressed, then pressure is released. It is important that you feel the pulse of the patient, make sure that you don't feel the capillaries of your fingers.
5. Pressure of the three examining fingers has to be uniform.
6. Pulse examination needs constant practice and much experience.

The state of *VĀYU* is indicated by the pulse felt with the INDEX.

The state of *PITTA* is indicated by the pulse felt with the MIDDLE FINGER.

The state of *KAPHA* is indicated by the pulse felt with the RING FINGER.

The basic character of the pulses:

Vāyu—movement of a snake or a leech 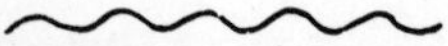

Pitta—movement of a crow, sparrow or frog 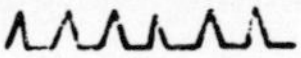

Kapha—movement of a swan or a peacock 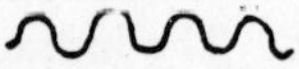

In a state of *sannipāta* (aggravation of all three *doṣas*) the pulse movement resembles a wood pecker: 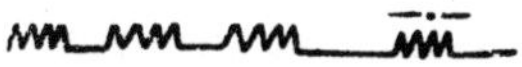

A healthy person's pulse is "like an elephant"=slow, steady and regular.

Regular pulse for 30 times always indicates good prognosis.

A pulse beating like this: 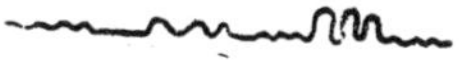 [1]
indicates bad prognosis.

While examining the pulse the following factors must also be taken into consideration:

+*Vāyu* (there is more *vāyu*) in: old age,
late afternoon,
late night,
2 hours after food,
during summer or beginning of rainy season.

+*Pitta* (there is more *pitta*) in: youth and middle age,
at noon,
at midnight,
during digestion of food
in the autumn.

+*Kapha* (there is more *kapha*) in: children,
the morning,
the evening (1st part of the night),
immediately after taking food,
the spring.

During pregnancy (bi-cardiac stage) there is a kind of double pulse: 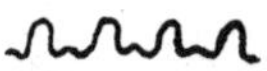

Wash your hands each time you have examined a pulse to avoid transmitting energies.

---

1. Very slow, soft below finger.

3. Urine-Examination (Mūtra-Parīkṣā)

Consult: FAM p. 94, BPA p. 42, Introd. p. 495.

Urine for examination should be collected in the morning after the patient got up from bed. The first flow of urine is discarded because it may contain extraneous material, the "middle-flow" is then collected in a clear glass vessel.

The actual examination should take place after sunrise. It involves two stages:

A) *The examination of the urine as it is*, i.e. its colour and degree of transparency are examined.

VĀYU predominance is indicated by pale yellow colour and, unctuous appearance.

PITTA predominance is indicated by more intensely yellow colour, reddish or blue colour and oil like appearance (like sesame oil).

KAPHA predominance is indicated by white and foamy appearance as well as a muddy look.

SĀNNIPĀTA condition (all 3 *doṣas* aggravated) is indicated by a blackish tinge of the urine.

INDIGESTION is indicated when the urine looks like lime juice or vinegar, water mixed with sandle wood paste (suspended material) or rice-wash.

FIRST STAGE OF FEVER is indicated by a smoky colour of the urine.

Relative variations of colour during the different seasons have to be taken into considerations. Thus during the rainy season the urine looks more whitish, while in summer it is more concentrated and therefore more intensely yellow.

B) *The examination of urine with the help of oil drops*

This examination takes place in the sun-light. The urine is kept in a clean wide-mouthed glass container and with the help of a dropper a little oil (sesame oil) is dropped into it. The spreading of the oil on the surface of the urine is then observed. Generally this takes place within 15 seconds. The following observations are significant:

I. If the oil spreads fast, the disease is cured relatively easily.

If the oil does not spread or spreads very slowly, cure of the disease is difficult.

If the oil settles down on the bottom of the glass, the disease is incurable.

II. The direction of movement of the oil is also observed. Movement to East—means quick recovery.

Movement to the South—indicates fevery conditions (or one to set in soon), recovery will be gradual.

Movement to the North—indicates freedom from disease or that the patient will be free from the disease very soon.

Movement to the West—indicates non-serious nature of the disease.

III. The resulting shape while the oil has spread out on the surface of the urine is taken into consideration.

Shape is interpreted as follows:

DIFFICULT CURE : plough, tortoise, buffalo, honeycomb, a man without head, arrow, sword, dagger staff or a cross road.

EASY CURE: swan, pond (◎), lotus, elephant, umbrella, gate, building.

Diseases are the result of actions in past lives, curses to the family or affictions by evil spirits are indicated by:

1. Holes like a sieve : 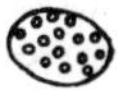
2. A full person.
3. Two heads.

VĀYU is indicated by a snake 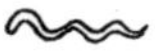

PITTA is indicated by an umbrella-like shape: 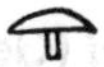

KAPHA is indicated by pearl-like shapes: ⁰₀⁰°

4. The Examination of Disease (Roga-Parīkṣā)

In the case of each disease the following points need carefull examination:

I. *Nidāna* (Etiology).
II. *Pūrva-Rūpa* (Premonitory Signs and Symptoms).
III. *Rūpa* (Actual Signs and Symptoms).
IV. *Upaśaya* (Exploratory Therapy).
V. *Samprāpti* (Pathogenesis).

These five steps are known as *pañca nidāna* (five-fold examination). They help the physician to arrive at the correct diagnosis of the disease. In descriptions of diseases in āyurvedic texts these five aspects are usually given in the beginning followed by the actual description of the treatment.

In the following we shall deal with each of the five aspects one by one.

I. Nidāna or Etiology

Etiology is the science of study of the causes of disease, both direct and predisposing, and the mode of their operation.

Causative factors of diseases are classified under 5 categories. (Frequently only 3 categories are mentioned, since the last two are actually included in the first three). The categories are:

1. *Prajñāparādha* (Intellectual blasphemy)
2. *Asātmyendriyārtha Saṁyoga* (Unwholesome contacts of senses with their objects)
3. *Kāla Pariṇāma* (Seasonal perversions)
4. *Karma* or *Saṁskāra* (Causative factors)
5. *Kṛmi* (Germs).

Now the categories in detail:

a. *Prajñāparādha* (Intellectual Blasphemy)

This includes perversions of the faculties of wisdom, patience and memory.

Prajñāparādha

Perversion of *Dhī* (wisdom) Acting against the laws of nature.	Perversion of *Dhṛti* (patience) Loss of patience, flaring up, acting at the wrong time.	Perversion of *Smṛti* (memory) Sins of omission.

→ *Karma* or *Saṁskāra* ←

Good or bad impressions of past lives.

b. *Asātmyendriyārtha Saṁyoga* (Unwholesome contact of senses with objects).

The tissue elements of the body are composed of the five basic *mahābhūtas*: *pṛthvī*, *jala*, *tejas*, *vāyu* and *ākāśa*, in different ratios. These tissue elements are continuously consumed by the *agnis* during the process of digestion and metabolism. Therefore, the *mahābhūtas* have to be replenished regularly.

The gross form of replenishment is done through food and drinks, the more subtle form of replenishment takes place through the sense organs:

Sound	Touch	Vision	Taste	Smell
Ākāśa	*Vāyu*	*Tejas*	*Jala*	*Pṛthvī*
Ears	Skin	Eyes	Tongue	Nose

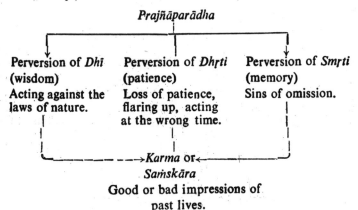

These contacts take place through germs, food, drinks, regimens. The "subtle halves" of the various *mahābhūtas* are real quanta of energy. It is not the anatomical ear, skin, eye, tongue or nose, which receive the quanta of energy, but they reach the soul through the mind (*manas*) and the intellect (*buddhi*). Therefore, the energy-quanta do not only replenish the regular loss of tissues through enzyme action, but also create an impact on the mind which regulates the functions of the body through the *doṣas*.

Perverted, excessive, or lack of contacts of the senses with their objects not only affects the tissues but also the mind resulting in the production of diseases.

c. *Kāla Pariṇāma* (Seasonal effects)

Because of climatic changes which are the result of solar, lunar and planetary effects, natural changes take place in the earth and its atmosphere as well as the human body. A certain change in the accumulation, aggravation or alleviation of *doṣas* during different seasons is normal and the biological processes in the body become adapted to these changes.

The individual (*piṇḍa*) is the replica of the Universe (*brahmāṇḍa*), and the effects of the macrocosm affect the individual (microcosm) continuously.

Here is a Table of the principal seasonal effects. (A=accumulation, Ag=aggravation, Al=alleviation, V=*vāyu*, *P*=*pitta*, K=*kapha*).

1. SUMMER →	K—Al	V—A
2. RAINY SEASON →	P—A	V—Ag
3. AUTUMN →	P—Ag	V—Al
4. WINTER (first part) →	P—Al	K—A
5. WINTER (later part)		
6. SPRING →	K—Ag	

Naturally in some zones there are only four seasons—summer, autumn, winter and spring.

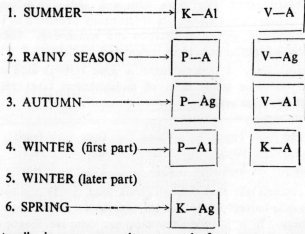

d. *Kāraṇa* (Cause)

Kāraṇas or causative factors are broadly classified into three categories:

1. *Nimitta,*
2. *Samavāyī,*
3. *Asamavāyī.*

Nimitta Kāraṇa are the necessary factors; for making a pot, vehicles or animals to carry the clay to the pottery. The skill of the potter, the implements for pottery etc. are only necessary during the preparation of the pot; afterwards their role is no longer required.

Analogically wrong diet, drinks and regimens constitute the *nimitta kāraṇas* of a disease.

Similar analogies can be made about weaving cloth.

Samavāyī Kāraṇa represents the basic matrix of any substance. For instance the clay needed for making a pot. *Doṣas, dhātus, agnis* and *srotas* are *samavāyī.*

Asamavāyī Kāraṇa is the putting together or joining of single entities. For instance, a pot consists of different parts, lower part, upper part, handle, spout, lid etc. If these joints are broken, the pot will cease to exist in its entirety.

Asamavāyī Kāraṇa is a kind of interaction in togetherness of single components. The interaction among the *doṣas* and *dhātus* for instance constitutes the *asamavāyī kāraṇa* of a disease.

Here is a Table of the *Kāraṇas*:

Kāraṇa

Samavāyī Kāraṇa	*Asamavāyī Kāraṇa*	*Nimitta Kāraṇa*
(Basic matrix of any substance)	(Putting together contact)	(Motive, efficient causes etc.)
Doṣa *Dhātu* *Agni* *Srota*	*Sammūrchana* (Conglomeration)	Transient: Food, Drink, Regimens Continuous: Germs

Nimitta Kāraṇas are divided into two categories:

1. Those that stop their activities after the disease is manifested.
2. Those that continue their activities even after the disease is manifested.

To the second category belong:

e. *Kṛmis* (Germs)

These multiply continuously and produce toxins which go on causing the disease after the later has manifested.

In healing we aim at stopping *nimitta kārṇas* and the destroying the *asamavāyī kāraṇas.*

II. Pūrva Rūpa (Premonitory Signs and Symptoms)

Premonitory signs and symptoms appear before the actual manifestation of the disease. They provide a clue to the diagnosis of the impending disease.

At this stage some diet restrictions as well as administration of medicines can avert the onset of the actual disease in many cases.

III. Rūpa (Actual Signs and Symptoms)

If the disease is not averted during the stage of *Pūrva Rūpa*, actual signs and symptoms (*Rūpa*) become manifest. All the actual signs and symptoms are related to :

1. The site of origin of a disease (*Udbhava Sthāna*).
2. The site of manifestation of a disease (*Adhiṣṭhāna*).
3. The path of transporation (*Sañcāra Mārga*).

Most of the signs and symptoms are associated with the site of manifestation of the disease.

Categories of *Rūpa* are :

(a) *Sāmānya* (general)
(b) *Viśiṣṭa* (specific)
(c) Invariable signs and symptoms
(d) Complications
(e) Other diseases
(f) Bad prognosis.

All actual signs and symptoms are related to the *doṣas, dhātus, agnis* and *srotas*. They are also connected with the site of origin (*udbhava sthāna*), the path of transportation (*sañcāra mārga*) and the site of manisfestation (*adhiṣṭhāna*) of the disease. For instance. Bronchial Asthma :

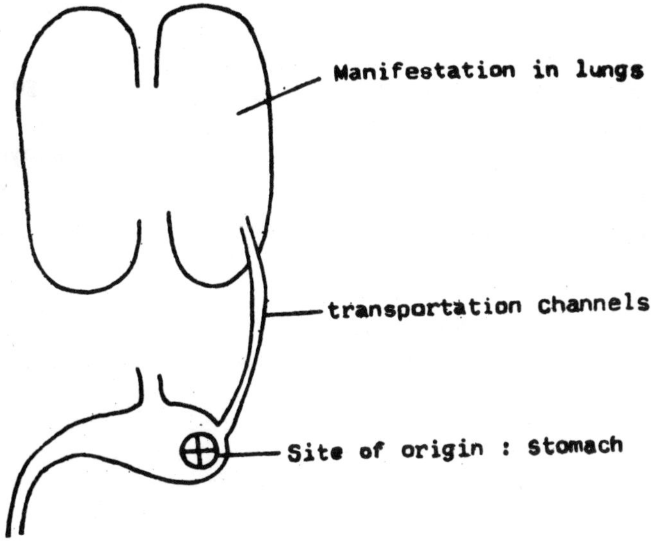

Rheumatism :

Colon	Joints
(site of origin)	(site of manifestation)

Most signs and symptoms, however, are connected with the site of manifestation of the disease.

Cardinal or specific signs and symptoms are called : *viśiṣṭa lakṣaṇa* (specific characteristics).

They are generally connected with the site of origin and the site of manifestation of the disease.

General signs and symptoms are called : *sāmānya lakṣaṇa* (general characteristics).

They play a secondary role in diagnosis. They indicate

to which extent the body is afflicted by the disease process, or also the organs afflicted by the disease as well as prognosis.

Symptomatic treatment is almost alien to āyurvedic medicine. It is the disease as a whole, including its site of origin as well as its site of manifestation which is taken into consideration for the choice of treatment.

The primary aim of treatment is to break the process of *samprāpti* (pathogenesis). For this reason not only the physical but also the mental set up of the patient is kept in view.

When symptoms become excessively painful, the āyurvedic physician resorts to symptomatic treatment in emergent situations.

IV. Upaśaya (Exploratory Therapy)

Exploratory Therapies are employed to ascertain the exact nature of a disease. There are, broadly speaking, eighteen categories of exploratory therapies on the basis of the drugs, diet and regimens which have opposite attributes or which have identical attributes but which actually work in the opposite manner to the cause of the disease, to the disease itself and/to both the cause and the disease.

Exploratory therapies are also important in ascertaining varieties of a disease.

Here follows a survey of the eighteen categories:

V. Samprāptī (Pathogenesis)

The manner with which a *doṣa* gets aggravated and moves through different channels or paths to produce a disease is called *samprāpti* or pathogenesis.

The process of manifestation of a disease proceeds through six different stages. Collectively these are called *kriyā kāla*.

I. *Sañcaya* (Accumulation). The *doṣa* gets accumulated in its own site. From this results:

II. *Prakopa* (Aggravation). In appropriate circumstances the level goes up, this leads to the third stage:

III. *Prasāra* (Spread). Because of increase in quantity, it does not remain confined to its own site. Involving paths of

Categories	*Drug*	*Diet*	*Regimen*
I. Having opposite attributes to cause. Example:			
Fever caused by *kapha* Fever caused by *vāyu*	dry ginger	meet, soup and rice	no sleep during day and keeping awake at night increases *vāyu*.
II. Having opposite attributes to disease. Example: Diarrhoea	bowel binding medicines (seeds of *Holarrhena anti-dysenterica* (*Indrayava*).	yoghurt.	Correct *udāvarta* (Upward movement abdominal wind).
III. Having opposite attributes to cause and disease. Example: Oedema caused by *vāyu*	*daśamūla* (group name of 10 drugs whose roots are used to cure oedema caused by *vāyu*).		
Sprue caused by *vāyu* and *kapha*		butter milk	
Sinusitis			avoid sleep during day which aggravates *kapha*. Remaining awake at night increases *vāyu*.

IV. Having similar attributes but working opposite to cause.		
Example:		
Inflammation caused by *pitta*	application of warming ointment	
V. Having similar attributes but working opposite to disease.		
Example:		
Vomiting	*madana* (*Randia dumetorum*)	Tenesmus (straining, especially to empty bowels or bladder)
Diarrhoea	Milk	
VI. Having similar attributes but working opposite to cause and disease.	*aguru* ointment (*Aquilaria agallocha*), which is hot in potency.	
Example:		
Burns		

Alcoholism	Takeg alcohol.	
Stiffness of thigh (*urus-tambha*) caused by *vāyu*.		Swimming.

Categories IV, V and VI are basic to homoeopathy.

An important basic rule to remember:

SESAME OIL	against	*VĀYU*
BUTTER	against	*PITTA*
HONEY	against	*KAPHA*

If *vāyu* is aggravated in its cold attribute : Give hot things.

If *vāyu* is aggravated in its ununctuous attribute : give unctuous thing.

transportation it spreads to other parts of the body. While moving through different channels, the aggravated *doṣa* gets lodged in a particular organ, this is called:

IV. *Sthāna Saṁśraya* (Location in a particular organ).

These first four categories are usually ignored by the patient. Only very careful patients would consult the physician at this time.

If the atmosphere and conditions in a paticular organ where the aggravated *doṣa* is now longed, are conducive to manifestation, the disease will now manifest. This stage is called:

V. *Vyakti* (Manifestation of the disease).

It then moves from generality to speciality, and specific varieties of the disease emerge. This stage is called:

VI. *Bheda* (Differentiation or varieties of the disease). At this stage the

Site of manifestation,
the Path of Transportation and
Site of Origin of the disease
have to be corrected simultaneously, otherwise the disease comes back.

It is during the last two stages (*Vyakti* and *Bheda* stages) that the patient usually consults the physician.

The *Samprāpti* determines the number or varieties of the disease (*saṁkhyā*), the attributes which are increased in the aggravated *doṣas* (*vikalpa*), the predominance of one over the other of the *doṣas* (*prādhānya*) in the manifestation of the disease, and the strength of the aggravated *doṣas* (*bala* & *kāla*).

2. Varieties or Types of Diseases

The three *doṣas* are the primary factors for the production of a disease. A disease may be caused by the aggravation of one of the *doṣas*, by aggravation of two *doṣas* simultaneously or by aggravation of all the three *doṣas* simultaneously. Since *doṣas* have certain attributes in common, aggravation of one *doṣa* may simultaneously lead to the aggravation of another *doṣa*.

Only the primarily aggravated *doṣa* which takes part in the *samprāpti* (pathogenesis) of the disease is taken into account while describing a disease.

In view of the just mentioned, there are seven varieties of *doṣa*-caused diseases:

I. The first three varieties are caused by aggravation of individual *doṣas*, either:

1. *Vāyu* (V), 2. *Pitta* (P), 3. *Kapha* (K).

II. The second three varieties involve the aggravation of two *doṣas* simultaneously:

4. *Vāyu-Pitta* (VP), 5. *Vāyu-Kapha* (VK),
6. *Pitta-Kapha* (PK) types.

III. The third group is characterised by aggravation of all the three *doṣas*. These types of diseases are called:

7. *Sannipāta* or *Sānnipātika* types of diseases. (S or VPK).

Some of the diseases known would fit into all the seven categories just mentioned. If we further consider, that the *doṣas* may aggravate in different proportions, the varieties of diseases are almost innumerable, but this is only of theoretical consideration. In practice we heal according to the standard rules regarding aggravation or *doṣas*.

Apart from the just mentioned *doṣic* varieties of diseases, there are a number of diseases not classified as V, P or K type of diseases.

Āsthmā, for instance, which according to āyurvedic concepts is of five kinds, does involve the three *doṣas* V, P and K, but the disease is treated differently through its own particular therapy. (We shall deal with āsthmā and its five varieties later). These special diseases are described on the basis of the following features:

1. Specific causative factors. (For instance like *kṛmija hṛdroga* = heart disease caused by germs, or *mṛd bhakṣaṇaja pāṇḍu* = anaemia caused by eating ordinary earth, mud, oven mud,

red ochre or chalk, which is an indication of lack of calcium).

2. On the basis of the path followed by the disease for its manifestation. For instance like *rakta pitta*—bleeding from various parts of the body, which may be upward (*ūrdhvaga*), downward (*adhoga*), or both ways simultaneously (*ubhayaga*). Effective medicines in this case are pearl, coral, the rhizome of water lillies and lotus.
3. On the basis of the afflicted viscera, (for instance like *kāmalā* (jaundice), which is either hepatic or pre-hepatic (*koṣṭhāśraya*) or obstructive (*śākhāśraya*).
4. On the basis of the shape of the affected part of the body. For instance like *kroṣṭuka śīrṣa* ("jackal-head"), a type of arthritis in which the knee looks like the head of a jackal.
5. On the basis of the stage of a disease. (For instance like *kumbha kāmalā*=chronic jaundice, in which due to the excess of bile the body looks almost greenish. Although this is only a stage of disease, it is treated in a special way.)

Regarding the stages of diseases we differentiate three stages:

1. *Āma* stage during this stage *āma* remains circulating in the body in large quantities. It is of different periods of duration.
2. *Pacyamāna* stage—this sets in, when the *āma* gets transformed gradually and is metabolised with drugs and regimens.
3. *Nirāma* stage—when the *āma* has been metabolised almost completely.

Āma should be corrected as early as possible, i.e. during the first stage. The disease gets fully cured only, when the site of origin becomes absolutely free from *āma*. But even during the last stage efforts to correct *āma* should not stop. *Āma* is present as long as the disease lasts. Because of this one of the synonyms of the term *roga* (disease) is *āmaya*.

3. Prognosis

Whatever the prognosis of a disease may be, the patient should be treated till the last breath. Even in terminal cases, at least the painful symptoms should be relieved. A physician should not give false assurances about cure. In case of incurability of the patient's condition, close relatives should be informed accordingly, not the patient himself, since otherwise he may die earlier than he is destined to. Patients with weak physical condition and weak willpower are difficult to cure. On the basis of their degree of curability, diseases are divided into three categories:

1. *Sukha sādhya* (of fortunate prognosis, i.e. curable or easily curable).
2. *Asādhya* (incurable or very difficult to cure).
3. *Yāpya* (palliable, a disease the patient has to live with.) Many obstinate skin diseases belong to this category.

Of course this scheme is always relative.

In making a prognosis the following conditions have to be taken into account:

1. The nature of the disease (V, K, P). V is often more difficult to treat, since it involves psychic elements as well.
2. The constitution of the patient. For instance V constitution + V disease is harder to cure.
3. The constitution, disease and season. For instance, V constitution + V disease + V season together make it more difficult to cure the disease.

Traditionally according to āyurveda for the prognosis of a disease a number of other factors are taken into consideration, for instance : the time of arrival of messengers contacting the physician, the condition of the physician when he is called to the patient, events on the way to the patients house (like behaviour of the wind, birds, animals etc., and events in the patients house (behaviour of relatives, animals etc.). Ref. BPA p. 441.

Āyurveda considers the span of life of a person to be predetermined, depending upon his actions during the past life, his activities during the present life and his environment, his attitudes etc. Birth under a particular constellation also determines the span of life.

By performance of virtuous acts, meditation and administration of rejuvenation therapies, the span of life can be increased and good health and vigour be maintained. Sinful life, however, may shorten the life span. Thus āyurveda, while basically recognising a predetermined span of life, also accepts the possibilities of its modification.

Life=Union of Body, Senses, Mind, Intellect and Soul.

These take up a new body when the old one wears out. The physiological process of death : "to become five". (The body breaks down into five *mahābhūtas*. The five sense organs withdraw, the *mahābhūtas* remain.

A verse to remember :

Vyādheḥ tattva parijñānam	To know disease from all aspects
vedanāyāḥ ca nigrahaḥ	to relive the pain of the patient
etat vaidyasa vaidyatvam	this is the physicianship of the physician
na vaidya prabhuḥ āyuṣaḥ	the physician is not the master of life.

4. Treatment

Treatment
is of two kinds

- Treatment of a HEALTHY PERSON for
  - Maintenance of POSITIVE HEALTH — *RASĀYANA* (Rejuvenation Therapy)
  - PREVENTION OF DISEASE — *VĀJIKARAṆA* (Aphrodisiacs)
- Treatment of a PATIENT who is already sick
  - Therapies leading to CURE OF DISEASE

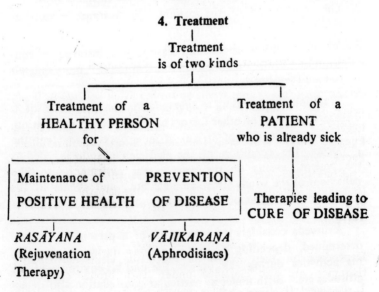

RASĀYANA
(Rejuvenation Therapy)
can be taken either

- when confined for treatment in a particular place
- or during work.

We shall now have a look at various therapies :

Therapies

- *Śodhana* (Elimination Therapies for prevention and cure)
  - K — Emesis
  - P — Purgation
  - V — Enema
- *Śamana* (Alleviation Therapies)
  - K — Honey
  - P — Butter, Ghee, *Āmalakī* (Use unsalted butter or a cup of milk. Butter alleviates P as well).
  - V — Sesame oil (or Castor oil if *āma* is present)

Enema is either *nirūha* (prepared with decoctions) or *anuvāsana* (prepared with oil etc.)

Along with the elimination and alleviation of *doṣas* it is necessary to promote the activities of the *agnis* (enzymes) responsible for digestion and metabolism. For this, the "Three Pungent Drugs" are useful : i.e. Ginger, Long Pepper and Black Pepper. We shall hear more about these at a later stage.

Besides the just mentioned therapies there is also *nasya* (inhalation therapy). Emesis, Purgation, the two types of Enema, and Inhalation are known collectively as "*pañca karma*" in āyurveda.

Categories of Therapies

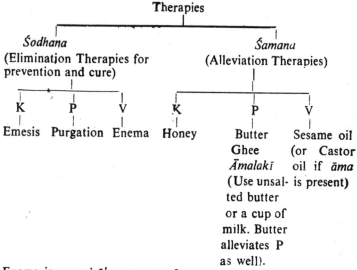

Depending on their effects on the tissue elements (*dhātus*), therapies are also classified under two broad categories, 1. *laṅghana* (fasting) which causes depletion of excessively accumulated tissue elements and 2. *bṛmhaṇa* (nourishing therapy) which promotes the quantity of depleted tissue elements. Four more categories supporting these processes are also described. These are *snehana* (oleation), *rukṣaṇa* (which produces a drying effects), *svedana* (fomentation) therapy which helps in the mobility of tissue elements and *stambhana* (which arrests the movement of excessively mobile tissue elements). These six categories together are known as *ṣaḍvidho-pakrama*. All drugs, diets, drinks and regimens prescribed in āyurvedic texts can be classified into these six categories.

Consult : FAM p. 112.

Here follows a systematic survey of the *ṣaḍvidho-pakrama*

LAṄGHANA (lightening, i.e. fasting)	*BṚMHAṆA* (nourishing)
RUKṢAṆA (drying)	*SNEHANA* (oleation)
SVEDANA (causing mobility through fomentation, this improves blood circulation and intestinal peristalsis)	*STAMBHANA* (arresting mobility, for instance to stop bleeding)

Consult : FAM 113-115.

Which types of medical recipes should be used? Four criteria are important.

The recipe should be :

1. *Vahu guṇa* (with many attributes), i.e. which cures many diseases. For instance one kind of medicine may serve against eczema, psoriasis and ringworm. Such broad-spectrum effect is important in case of doubtful diagnosis.
2. *Vahu kalpa* (the recipe should be capable of being used in the form of many pharmaceutical preparations. For instance as an infusion, tincture, with honey, wine etc.)
3. *Yogya* (lit. serviceable, fit, adapted). It should not have unpleasant side-effects and be free from toxicity. It is no use to cure one disease and cause another. Iatrogenetic diseases are to be avoided.

4. *Sampanna* (That which is part of the culture of a people). For instance Hindus don't eat beef, Muslims don't eat pork and don't drink wine, and so forth. Āyurveda respects different religious and social customs. Don't administrate medicines contrary to the patients' religious and social convictions.

In treatment take care simultaneously of :

1. The Site of Origin of a disease.
2. The Spreading of a disease.
3. The Site of Manifestation of a disease.

as far as this is possible at all time.

For medicinal use we have at our disposal:

1. Drugs, Diet, Drinks and Regimens. Drugs can be of vegetable origin and in some cases also of animal origin. Mostly plant and animal substançes are used, but there are also mineral preparations. During the later Buddhist period minerals became more popular in āyurvedic medicine than before, specially since surgery was prohibited during this period. Characteristic for mineral preparations are :

   1. fast action, 2. almost complete tastelessness,
   3. their administration in very small dose.

2. The use of Instruments, Equipments, Alkalies, Cauterization, application of Leeches, Bees etc.
3. The use of *Mantras* or Psychic Therapy.

5. Preparation-Methods of Medicines

Pharmaceutical processes adopted for different categories of medicines are as follows :

a. *Juice (svarasa)*. The juice is pressed from plants, generally it is cold-pressed. In some cases hard leaves have to be cooked first over fire in the form of a mud bolus.
Example : *Kākamācī* (*Solanum nigrum*=Black Nightshade) is

used against various liver disorders, like infantile cirrhosis. The juice has a bland taste and is given to children with honey or milk.

Kumārī (*Aloe vera*), is given to girls during early puberty against dysmenorrhea, hormonal unbalance and against liver. disfunction in both sexes. The juice has a bitter taste. Usually the plant is first steam boiled, the juice is then squeezed out.

Bilva (*Aegle marmelos Corr.*), a plant which is also used in *Śiva-pūja*, has bitter-astringent taste. For extracting the juice a bolus of mud is made, the leaves are heated in this, the bolus is then broken and the juice squeezed out.

In case of diabetes, this juice is taken for 10 days; after this the blood sugar level remains, but the sugar level in the urine is reduced, a feeling of happiness results.

Or one leaf  like this is taken twice per day. This is not useful in children's diabetes. If the blood sugar should be completely normalised : take it for 6 months.

b. *Powder* (*cūrṇa*). Plants are dried in the shade and then powdered. Certain plants may also be exposed to the sun while drying. Powder only when completely dry, otherwise there may be a fungus. Store in a dry place in a dry container well closed. Remains active for 1 year. Often different powders are mixed.

Example : *Eclipta alba* is a plant often used in hair oil, but it is also taken internally, since it corrects the function of the liver. To this powder, the powder of *Picorrhiza Kurroa* is added along with the powdered rocksalt. The salt has to be powdered separately and then added.

Some of the more woody plants can only be ground with the help of some kind of machine. For instance *Glycyrrhiza glabra* (liquorice) has a hard root. The powder of this root is not only used as a laxative, but also in cases of rheumatism and as a rejuvenating medicine. (For the latter purpose the root is also boiled in milk).

c. *Infusion* (*phāṇṭa*). These are mostly hot infusions of herbs in water, the classical herb-teas, mint, rose, jasmin etc. The herbs are steeped for a few minutes and then the infusion is strained. Always cover while steeping.

d. *Decoction* (*kvātha*). For this the drug is boiled in water. According to the hardness of the drug, either four, eight or sixteen times of water is added and then boiled till about 1/4 remains. The decoction is then filtered and the filtrate used medically. Sometimes various things are added, like butter, honey (cold) or oils.

e. *Paste* (*kalka*).

f. *Milk preparation.* (*kṣīra pāka*). For instance liquorice boiled with milk. Generally one part of the drug is mixed with 8 part milk and 32 parts of water and boiled till one fourth remains. The whole is then filtered and the filtrate taken after adding sugar etc.

g. *Cold infusion.* (*śīta kaṣāya*). The drug is soaked in water and kept overnight. Next morning it is filtered and the filtrate taken after adding sugar, honey etc. Generally one spoon per tumbler of water is used.

Example : *Triphalā* (Three Fruits) is used like this. *Triphalā* means: *Harītakī* (*Terminalia chebula*)+*Bibhitakī* (*Terminalia belerica*)+*Āmalakī* (*Emblica officinalis*) mixed in powder form. One teaspoon is mixed with a tumbler of water, the next morning this is filtered through a cloth. Half of the liquid is used for washing the eyes, the rest is taken internally, after adding a little honey. It is astringent. *Triphalā cūrṇa* promotes power of resistance, it is added to many āyurvedic preparations for this reason, apart from being a medicine for a variety of disorders. We shall come back to *Triphalā* at a later stage.

h. *Linctus or Jam* (*avaleha lehyam Pāka, prāśa or khaṇḍa*). This is a typical āyurvedic preparation, of which perhaps the excellent tonic known as *Cyavana prāśa* is perhaps the best example. *Cyavana prāśa* is rich in *Āmalakī* (*Emblica officinalis*), which is useful in treating chronic diseases of the lungs like chronic bronchitis and tuberculosis. *Cyavana prāśa* is widely used for cough and respiratory tract ailments.

i. *Medicated oils* (*taila*), are oils containing herbal extracts. They are used for the hair, the head, for massage, enemas etc. We shall hear later about various recipes.

j. *Medicated ghee* (*ghṛta*). For instance *Triphalā Ghṛta*, which is *Triphalā* boiled in butter or ghee. These medicines are mainly for P and V disorders, if the liver is good and if there is no bad digestion.

k. *Alcoholic preparations* (*āsava and ariṣṭa*). In the case of *ariṣṭa* the drug is first of all boiled, while when making an *āsava*, the drug is simply added. Both are actually varieties of herbal wines, prepared by natural fermentation with yeast. The maximum alcohol percentage is about 15.

All the drugs, juices etc. are fermented in a suitable container. In the old days an earthen pot was used, the inside border of which was smeared with a little turmeric powder and ghee to avoid that the whole turned sour. The pot is then kept for about a month. Many different recipes of this kind are given in the texts, to which we shall come at a later stage.

l. *Pills or tablets* (*vaṭi or guṭikā*).

m. *Large size pills* (*modaka*).

n. *Scale preparations* (*parpaṭi*). These are generally prepared by pouring a substance on a leaf. For instance, mercury and sulphur are put into a spoon, melt through heat, then pour over a banana leaf It forms a scale.

o. *Medicines prepared by sublimation* (*kūpīpakva rasāyana*). This means literally: rejuvenating agent prepared in a glass bottle.

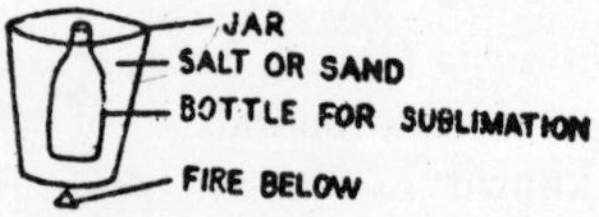

The mouth of the bottle is kept open in the beginning, later it is closed. In this way for instance sulphur gets sublimated.

Don't let it clog. After some time some peculiar colour becomes visible above, seal, reduce heat, keep for 12 hours. Break bottle to obtain sublimate.

p. *Bhasma* (calcination) *of metals, gems, plants and animal products.* Metals and minerals are invariably used in *bhasma* form. Many *bhasmas* are highly complex preparations. Since many metals and minerals are toxic when given in their ordinary state, they have to be made non-toxic, and to be brought to the state in which they can be absorbed easily. Gold, for instance, will not get assimilated if given to a patient in the form of filings or leaf, rather it will act as a poison. Through a special process we can make the gold non-toxic and transform it into a marvellous medicine. This is done as follows : Gold is heated till glowing, it is then dipped seven times after each heating into:

1. Sesame oil
2. Butter milk
3. Urine of a Virgin cow
4. Vinegar
5. *Kulattha* (*Dalichos biflorus*), a pulse type. It is first boiled.

Bhasmas involve oxidation processes. Iron given in raw form would be quite useless, since it would cause only constipation. The āyurvedic *bhasma* preparations on the other hand, do not in the least cause any digestive problems but goes to the blood quickly to increase hemoglobin.

The preparation of metals usually beings with *śodhana* (purification). This is not only removal of chemical impurities but the process of making them non-toxic. This is followed by *māraṇa* (killing) and by *amṛtī karaṇa* (the making of nectar) out of them. These highly complex preparations are described in the separate section called *Rasa Śāstra*, which is part of the āyurvedic scriptures. Some of these preparations may take even years to prepare.

For mercury, there are 18 kinds of purifications (18 stages).

1. *Svedana*: it is added to a sour gruel and boiled.
2. *Mardana*: trituration.

3. *Mūrchana*: fainting, breaks into small globules.
4. *Utthāpana*: Sublimation.
5. *Pātana*: upward sublimation, distillation and downward  sublimation. For the last variety it is smeared in a pot, heat is then applied and it falls down. Then three more steps are to follow. After these eight steps mercury becomes fit to be used in ordinary recipes. For special recipes to prevent and cure diseases (*deha vāda*) and alchemy (*dhātu vāda*) ten more steps are to follow. *Deha-vāda* is supposed to make the body light. Nāgārjuna used it for flying.

   All these kind of recipes constitute the alchemical secrets of āyurvedic medicine, we shall return to these at the proper time.

q. *Piṣṭi* (reducing gems to fine power by triturating with juice of drugs.)

r. *Collyrium* (*añjana*), these are special preparations for the eyes. For instance, Antimony powder, or lead oxide, or the soot from a lamp burning with caster oil which is covered by a copper vessel is used as the base. There are many kinds of collyrium.

s. *Elongated pills* (*vartī*).

t. *Poṭṭalī* (preparations made out of metals etc. by cooking them in the form of small bolus).

u. *Arka* (preparations made by distillation). These contaln essential oils and often are stronger alcoholic preparations, since ordinarily fermented preparations cannot have more than 15% alcohol because fermentation stops at this percentage.

Some of the plant preparations are also more complicated to prepare.

Examples : *Aconite*. This is used for the treatment of fever and pain. There are different varieties of *Aconite Aconitum feroxum*, *Aconitum Chasmanthum* and *Aconitum nepallus* are the most commonly used varieties.

The plant has 2 roots : 

These 2 roots are taken together, since one counteracts the poison of the other, they are complimentary to each other. The outer bark of the roots is scarped out and roots cut into pieces and kept for 7 days in cow's urine, preferably virgin cow's urine, and then taken out. This works as a cardiac tonic without being depressive.

Strychnus Nux Vomica. The outer layer of the *nux vomica* is taken out and soaked in cow's milk for 21 days. Then it looses its poisonous character but remains bitter. This is tonic for the nervous system.

6. Names of Recipes and Medicines

Most of the recipes described in āyurvedic texts have a name. The names are given on the basis of the following:

1. *On the basis of the first drug mentioned in the recipe.* This is very common.

   Example : *Kumāri-Āsava.* A self generated alcoholic preparation of *Aloe vera*, Molasses and several other drugs. It is used to promote digestion, proper functioning of the liver and for female disorders. *Pippali Āsava*, which is prepared from long pepper+12 other ingredients.

2. *Named after the original propounder.*

   Example : *Cyavana-Prāśa.* This is named after the Saint Cyavana. *Prāśa* means jam, linctus or *lehyam.*

3. *On the basis of the proportion of drugs used in the recipe.*

   Example : *Pañca Kola* (which means: 5 units of 12 grams, so 5 units of 12 grams of different drugs are used).

4. *On the basis of the number of drugs used in the recipe.*

Example : *Triphalā* which is a combination of the three drugs *Harītakī, Bibhitakī and Āmalakī* already mentioned previously.

5. *On the basis of the therapeutic effect of the recipe.*

Example : *Śvāsa Kuṭhāra* (the axe which cuts the tree of āsthmā).

Makara Dhvaja (a potent sex stimulant named after the God of sex).

Mṛtyuñjaya Rasa (Medicine to overcome death). For serious types of fever.

7. Diet

Suitable diet is very important for positive health and for prevention of disease. It has been said : "Without proper diet, medicines are of no use, and with proper diet, medicines are of no use (are unnecessary)." In the first case the disease will not get cured in spite of the use of suitable medicines. In the second case proper diet by itself may cure the disease. The idea reminds of Hippocrates who said that food should be our medicine and medicine our food.

Diets work through:

1. Taste (*rasa*): These are related to the five *mahābhūtas*.
2. Potencies (*vīrya*), which are 2 or 8 in number, as we had seen previously.
3. Taste after digestion (*vipāka*) which is either sweet, sour or pungent.
4. *Prabhāva* (specific action), which is produced on the basis of 20 *guṇas* (qualities or attributes).

Contradictory food is to be avoided. Contradictory are for instance:

ghee and honey in equal quantity,
alkalies taken for a very long time,
salt taken for a very long time,
milk and fish together,
honey in hot drinks.
Contradictory regimen: for instance sleeping during the day when there is *āma* formation.

CHAPTER THREE

The Drugs

1. HARĪTAKĪ

Different varieties of *Harītakī* are described in āyurvedic texts, and the size of the fruit of this tree, which is used in medicine, varies. The tropical tree, which is found growing at altitudes upto 650 m, possesses a great trunk, thick leaves, yellowish flowers and blackish-yellow or blackish-brownish fruits.

The fruit is used in medicine, the seed is taken out and the whole pulp is then used. Modern Western books of botanic medicine rarely mention this species, but in ancient works *Harītakī* is dealt with at great length. Tabernaemontanus in his famous Herbal of 1731, describes the species and its virtues at length. Three etchings from his work are given in page 85.

Consult : FAM 158.

Tabernaemontanus describes A as large or black-brown myrobalan,
B as Indian or black Myrobalan,
C as yellow myrobalam.

The blackish-brown variety is the most important.

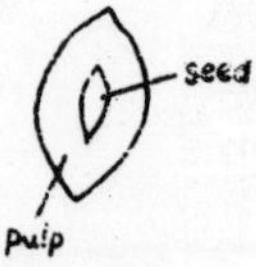

Bot. Name : *Terminolia chebula*

Fam. : Combretaceae.

Engl. : Chebulic Myrobalan, True Myrobalan Gall-Nut, Ink-Nut.

German : Groβ oder Schwarz-Braune Myrobalanen.

Chinese : Ho-tzu.

Rasa : *Harītakī* has 5 of the 6 tastes. Only the saline taste is missing. (Only three botanical species have 5 tastes, the other being Garlic (*lasuna*) and *Emblica officinalis* (*āmalakī*).

Aſchenfarb Myrobalanen.
Myrobalani Emblicæ.
Groß oder ſchwartzbraun Myrobalanen.
Myrobalani chebulæ.

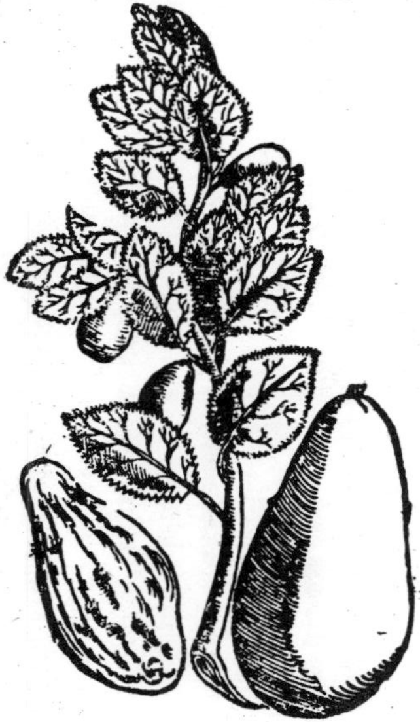

Indianiſch oder ſchwartz Myrobalanen.
Myrobalani Indicæ.

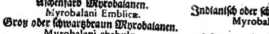

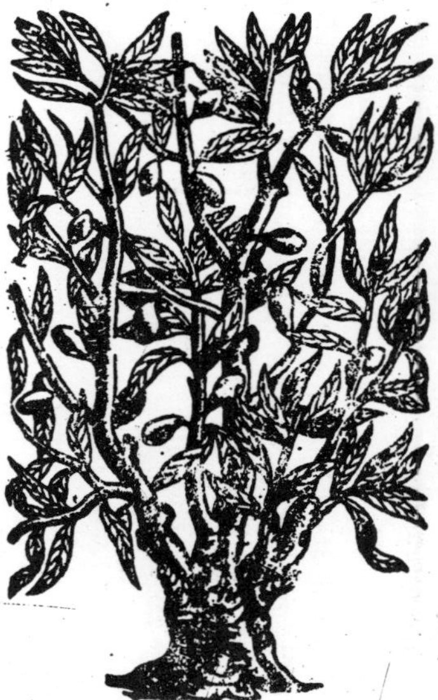

Geel Myrobalanen.
Myrobalani flavæ, citrinæ, luteæ.

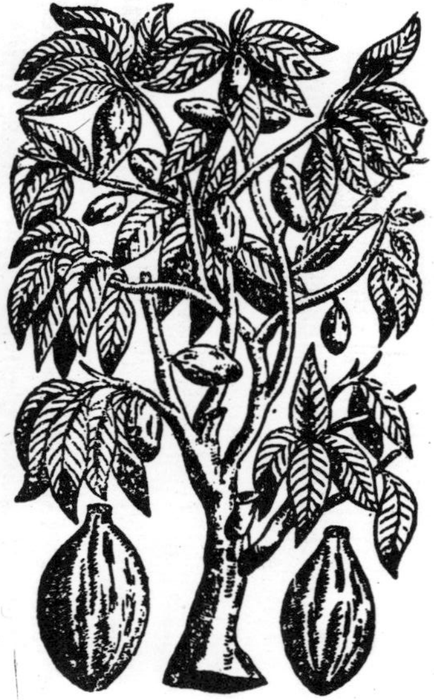

The 5 tastes explain some of its virtues:

	Sweet	Sour	Pungent	Bitter	Astringent
alleviates :	—V	—V	—K	—P —K	—K —P

This survey shows that *Harītakī* is excellent for curing V, P and K excess.

***Vīrya* : Hot.**

***Vipāka* : Sweet**

Action : Anabolic

***Harītakī* is one of the very best general tonics, and probably the best known medicinal species of āyurvedic pharmacology. Its name is related to *hṛ* (to take away), because it takes away diseases.**

In Tibetan it is known as the "King or the Best of Medicines" (*smun-mchog rgyal-po*). In āyurveda it is compared to the care and usefulness of a mother, except that unlike a real mother, it never becomes angry.

Harītakī promotes long life, rejuvenates, stimulates enzymatic action in case of obstruction of channels (enzymes are activated by its hot character). It helps in the metabolic transformation of *āma*.

Harītakī grown in cold climate is rejuvenating. The variety grown in hotter climate is more of a purging type. A very dark small variety is contraindicated in pregnancy. It enters into many medicines of the āyurvedic formulary. When taken as it is :

In summer it is taken with a little jaggery (molasses),
during the rainy season it is taken with a little rock-salt,
in autumn it is taken with a little brown sugar,
in early winter it is taken with a little ginger powder,
during the later winter it is taken with a little long pepper and
during spring it is taken with a little honey.

A small piece with a little salt before meals will avoid constipation.

Harītakī is also excellent for eyesight and skin diseases, further for rheumatism and diabetes.

An example of an äyurvedic recipe containing *Harītakī* is :

Agastya Harītakī or *Agastya Rasāyana*, a famous tonic.

This formula was created by the sage Agastya, the original propounder of the Siddha System of Medicine. (See FAM p. 119).

One thousand mature dried *Harītakī* fruits are put into a cloth bundle which is then boiled in a pot containing 20 different medicinal drugs. The *Harītakī* pulp is then freed from fibre and seed. The rest of the decoction together with the pulp and a little ghee is then made into a kind of jam.

We shall return to *Harītakī* many times during our course.

Use in Chinese medicine : *Ho-tzu* is considered to have warming properties and bitter sour and peppery taste. It stimulates the intestines, strengthens the lungs, lowers excessive energy output, is used against chronic cough and hoarse voice, chronic diarrhoea and dysentery, prolapse of the rectum, intestinal flatus, leukorrhea, seminal emission and excessive perspiration.

Use in Western medicine: Tabernaemontanus mentions *Harītakī* as a purging species, and as a "blessed medicine" because of its gentle action and its capacity to strengthen the heart, the stomach and the liver and, in fact, the entire organism. It liberates the system of "burnt black bile" and cures melancoly and depression. It is favourable in all diseases which have their origin in "excessive melancoly", such as cancer, many types of skin diseases, depression, heart trembling etc. The species purifies and drives away phlegm and slime through passing stool. It also sharpens the eye sight and all the senses. Together with honey or sugar the species strengthens the heart. Serves as an appetizer, digestive, sharpens the senses and gives clear eyesight, good against excessive thirst, and an excellent strengthener of the brain and the nerves.

No wonder that *Harītakī* is considered such a marvellous over-all tonic, Buddhas, are represented with this fruit in one of their hands.

2. BIBHĪTAKĪ

This type of myrobalan grows at heights up to 1000 m, in dry regions. It gives much fruit and is found wild in many parts of India. Some roads in Delhi are lined with this species, a big tree.

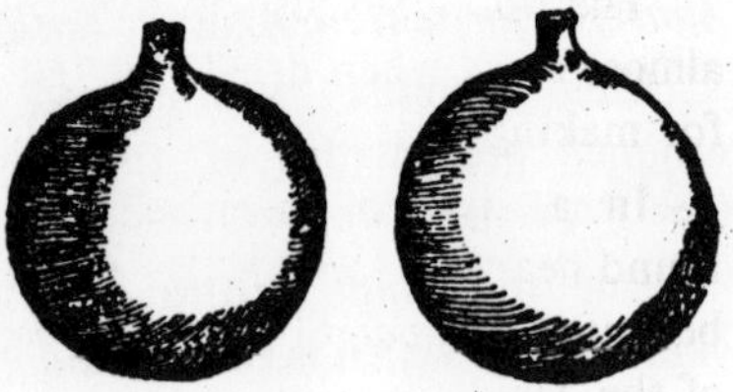

Myrobalani Bellericæ ſiccæ.

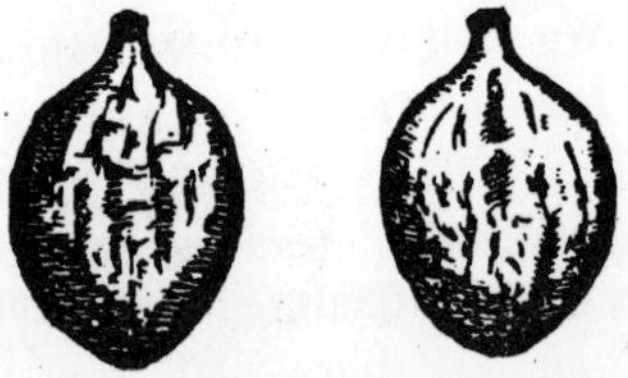

Bot. Name : *Terminalia belerica*
Fam.: Combretaceae.
German: Grüne bellerische Myrobalanen.
Rasa: Astringent.
Vīrya: Hot.
Vipāka: Sweet.
Action : Alleviates KPV.
Anabolic.
In case of: Bronchitis (expectorant)
Āsthmā (seed-pulp).
Vomiting (as a preventive specially during pregnancy)
Inflammatory conditions anywhere in the body.
Allergies (acts as an anti-allergic. Mixed with turmeric it is used against āsthmā and skin diseases).
Constipation.
Colics (it has a little narcotic effect)

It is good for eyesight, hair, and for diseases. *Rasa*, *Rakta*, *Māṁsa* and *Medas*, and also for reducing weight.

Use in Western medicine : according to Tabernaemontanus, mainly as a cleansing tonic.

3. ĀMALAKĪ

This tree of the Euphorbiaceac family grows in tropical, sub-tropical and temperate climate upto a height of about 1500 m above sea level.

The cultivated variety has large fruits and less fibre in the pulp, while the fruits of the wild variety are smaller.

The fruit consists of five segments or lobes, it becomes almost black when dried. It is also used as a vegetable and for making jams.

In a stylised form, as a stone sculpture, the fruit is often found near the top of the towers of North Indian temples, because the *āmalakī* tree is supposed to have been the first tree of the Universe.

The entire tree is used in medicine, although the fruits are by far the most important part used.

Myrobalani Fmblicæ.

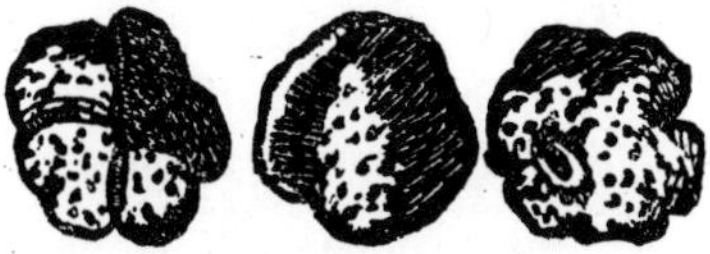

An etching from Tabernaemontanus famous Herbal 1731.

Bot. Name : *Emblica officinalis*

Fam. : Euphorbiaceae

German : Aschenfarb Myrobalanen

Rasa : Sweet, Sour, Pungent, Bitter and Astringent (no Saline taste)

Vīrya : Cooling

Vipāka : Sweet

Action : *Anabolic*

Effect : Sour alleviates V. Sour generally aggravates P. *Āmalakī* is an exception to this rule. Sweet & Cold alleviate P.
Astringent, Bitter and Pungent taste alleviate K.

Āmalakī is rich in vitamin C, which is thermostable, it has a fixed oil and an essential oil as well as tannin.

Āmalakī is an excellent plant for rejuvenation, as nourishment and as a tonic. It is good for eyesight and for the hair (boiled with sesame oil which is greasy, or with coconut oil, which is not greasy).

Āmalakī is used against : Skin diseases
Piles (acts as a laxative and corrects liver function). Diabetes (*Āmalakī* and Turmeric for long treatment, of at least 1 year, no immediate effect).
Heart disease.
Anaemia (together with iron *bhasma*).
Haemorrhages.
Diarrhoea.
Jaundice.
Bronchitis,
Asthma.

For good eyesight : *Āmalakī* can be boiled in cow's ghee (*āmalakī ghṛta*), this preparation is good for eyesight in case of progressive myopia. Also the powder of *āmalakī* soaked in water overnight can be applied to the eyes.

Āmalakī is part of many medicinal formulae of Āyurveda, together with *Harītakī* and *Bibhitakī* it forms the famous *Triphalā* preparations.

Use in Western medicine : Purifies the stomach and intestinal tract of foul phlegm and tonifies the stomach. Strengthens brain, heart, nerves and liver, against heart trembling, improves appetite, reduces excessive heat and quenches the thirst. Tabernaemontanus mentions that various kinds of jams are made from this fruit with the addition of cinnamon, cardamom, xylaloe, crocus etc.

4. TRIPHALĀ

Triphalā (three fruits) is a combination of *Āmalakī*, *Bibhitakī* and *Harītakī*. *Triphalā* can be prepared in various ways, as a powder, as a jam, in the form of drinks and so forth.

The preparation is given for the strengthening and rejuvenation of the tissues. *Āma* formation is neutralized by strengthening the *agnis* (enzymes). Apart from being superb tonic, *triphalā* is also used specifically for asthma, bronchitis and *meha* (obstinate urinary disorders, including diabetes).

5. ŚUṆṬHĪ

Ginger is a perennial, creeping plant with a thick tuberous rhizome, which produces an erect annual stem 60-120 cm tall. The lanceolate leaves are 1-2 cm wide and 15-30 cm long. Flowers in spikes are greenish marked with purple on long peduncles.

The plant is native to South East Asia, but spread to many tropical countries, it grows upto altitudes of 1500 m.

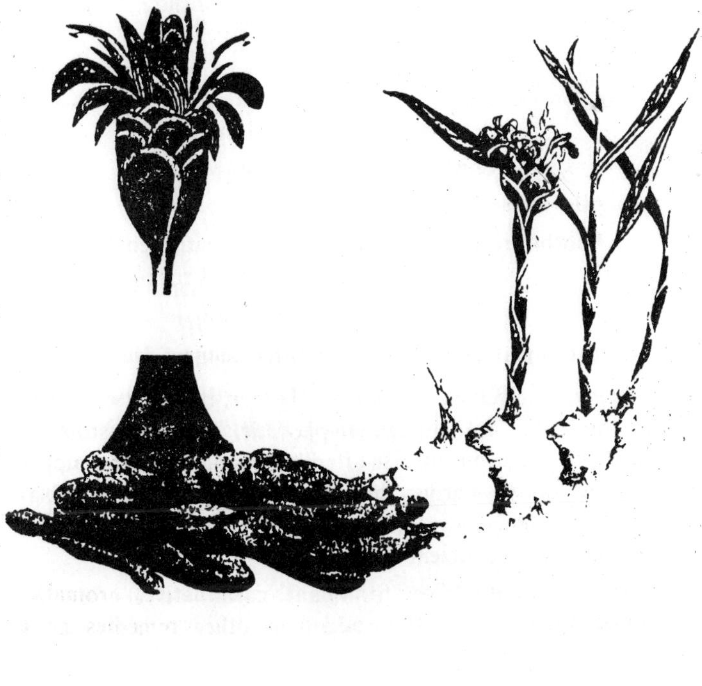

Propagated from rhizome cuttings, planted on rich, well drained loam.

Ginger contains potassium oxalate, essential oil (3%) comprising comphene, phelandrene, zingiberine, gingerol, resin and starch.

Bot. Name : *Zingiber officinale.*
Fam. : Zingiberaceae.
Engl. : Ginger.
German : Ingwer.
Chinese : Chiang, Kan-Chiang, Cheng-Kiang (Mand.), Sang-keung (Cant.).
Arabic : Amomum Zerumbeth.
Rasa : Pungent.
Vīrya : Hot.
Vipāka : Sweet.

Action : Carminative (in case of flatulence, colics)
Cardiac tonic
Digestive stimulant
Constipation (dry ginger is very useful)
Chronic Arthritis

Anorexia (juice + honey, one spoon of each, as a delicious appetizer and digestive).
Ginger can also be taken with salt.

Alleviates V and K.

Another recipe : put ginger pieces into lemon juice, keep in the sun, add rock-salt and a little sugar or honey.

Ginger is part of Tri-Kaṭu (the three pungent drugs)

Use in Chinese medicine : Of pungent flavour, it increases *Yang.* Chases the cold, anti-emetic, diaphoretic, increases stomach and intestinal secretion; in case of energy rising into the upper part of the body; warms the central region, used in moxa. Against *Yang* deficiency, slow pulse, cold extremities, moist coughs, diarrhoea, deficient-cold stomach/spleen.

Use in Western medicine : Stimulant, carminative, aromatic, sialogogue, anti-emetic. Often added to other remedies as a general tonic or stimulant. Against flatulent colic, dyspepsia, added to purgatives to prevent gripping.

"Carries the forces of fire into the earth" (Pelikan).

6. MARICA

Black pepper is a perennial climbing shrub with glossy, strongly nerved ovate-oblong leaves upto 18 cm long and 12 cm wide on 2 cm petioles. Flowers on spikes are white; the fruit is yellow at first, then red, a small globe of 6 mm.

A native of South India, it now grows in all tropical

Grüne bellerische Myrobolanen.
Myrobalani Bellericæ recentes.

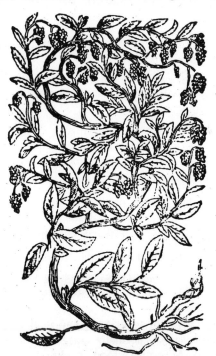

countries where there is water. It requires shade and high humidity, In South India it is often seen growing up on coconut trees. Historically speaking, it is the most important spice.

White pepper is from the same species, only the black coat of the fruit is taken off. The dried, unripe fruits of this plant are used. Constituents are a volatile oil (2 5%) comprising the alkaloids piperine, piperidine and chavicine; a yellow compound piperettine, traces of hydrocyanic acid, resins and starch.

Bot. Name : *Piper nigrum.*
Fam. : Piperaceae.
Engl. : Black pepper.
German : Schwarzer Pfeffer.
Chinese : Hu-chiao, Hu-tsiao (Mand.), Wou-tsiu (Cant.)
Greek : πεπεϱi.
Arabic : Fulfel or Filfel.
Rasa : Pungent.
Vīrya : Hot.
Vipāka : Pungent (not sweet like the other pungent drugs).
Action : Reduces K, V and fat.
Stimulates digestion.
For Heart Diseases.
Bronchitis (Expectorant).
Tonsilitis (which is usually associated with constipation), as a disinfectant.
Sinusitis.
as an appetiser,
against colic pains,
intestinal parasites,
many diseases of the head.

Black pepper stimulates the enzymes in the digestive tract, the liver and the tissue elements. It is dominated by ***agni-mahābhūta***, its action is catabolic.

It is a powerful drug for reducing K and it also reduces V. (this is an exception, since normally pungent-bitter-astringent tastes aggravate V). Mixed with food, drinks, honey or milk, it regulates digestion. While chillies can irritate the stomach, black pepper does not.

Taken for 6 months regularly it reduces the tendency to accumulate fat in the body. (1 teaspoon per day). It is good for heart diseases, specially coronary thrombosis, (it helps in downward movement of wind, therefore it releases the heart.)

Black pepper also helps as an expectorant. It increases the watering from the nose and later dries up phlegm. Creates a hostile atmosphere against intestinal parasites.

Use with care where there is aggravation of pitta (*pitta* type of sleeplessness and headaches). Use with care also in case of gastric or duodenal ulcers.

Marica is part of *Tri-Kaṭu* (the three pungent drugs).

Use in Chinese medicine : *Hu-chiao* has warming properties, is acrid to taste, warms central organs and dispels cold, eliminates abdominal distension and alleviates pain, used against cold, cold stomach, abdominal fullness, cold energy predominance, "*Yin* cold", abdominal pain, food poisoning. Clears excessive *Yin* and troubles of moisture, arrests vomiting, anti-mucus, anti-parasitic, chases water. Tonifies the *Yang* of the kidneys, acts upon lung and three-heater meridians.

Use in Western medicine : According to the classical tradition, pepper warms and dries in the third degree, it opens up, resolves and reduces fat. According to Tabernaemontanus pepper is warm and dry in the fourth degree, it is penetrating, opening, dividing, eliminates phlegm and "makes thin".

Black pepper is used as a stomachic, carminative, aromatic stimulant, antibacterial, diaphoretic. It stimulates gastric secretion, mucous membranes and part of the nervous system, raises body temperature.

Widely used as a spice.

7. PIPPALI

Long pepper grows mainly in India, Java and the Philippines. The unripe spikes are gathered when still green, this way they are hotter than when ripe. The fruit is somewhat greyish in colour with a weak aromatic odour and a pungent fiery taste, particularly after taste. It contains piperine, a soft green resin, a burning acridity and volatile oil, which is responsible for its aromatic odour.

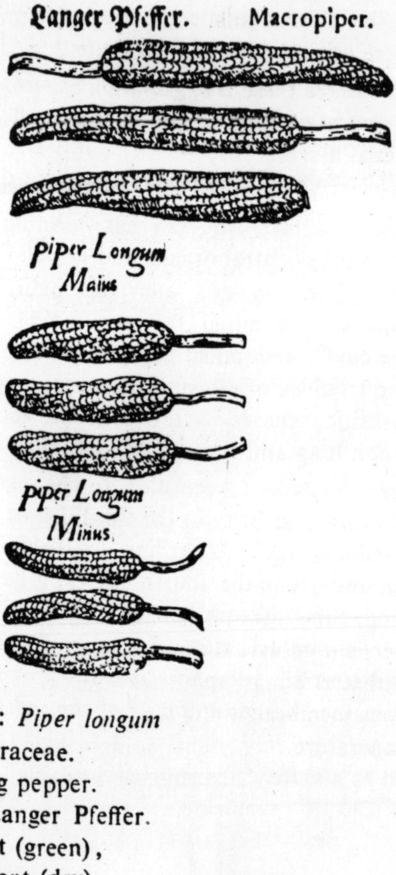

Bot. Name : *Piper longum*
Fam. : Piperaceae.
Engl. : Long pepper.
German : Langer Pfeffer.
Rasa : Sweet (green),
Pungent (dry).
Vīrya : Hot.
Vipāka : Sweet.
Action : Carminative.
Digestive.
Stimulant.
Emetic.

Rejuvenating.
Alleviates K and V.
Used against : Fevers, Spleen complaints,
Spleen disorders.
Skin diseases.
Rheumatism.
Asthma.
Diabetes.
Piles.
Tuberculosis.
Bronchitis.

Long paper is part of *Tri Kaṭu* (the three pungent drugs),

Use in Western medicine : Most classical texts make little difference between the use of black pepper and long pepper, except that long pepper is considered more gentle "because of its excessive moisture" (Tabernaemontanus).

8. TRI KAṬU

Ginger, Black Pepper and Long Pepper mixed together are known as *Tri-Kaṭu* in Āyurveda, i.e. as "the three pungent drugs".

They stimulate the *agnis* (enzymes) very well because of their *tejas-mahābhūta* nature. Although Black Pepper is pungent in *Vipāka*, Ginger and Long Pepper are sweet in *Vipāka*, therefore *Tri-Kaṭu* remains sweet in *Vipāka*.

Tri-Kaṭu is a very important combination in Āyurveda, which is used as a stimulant, carminative, against cold etc. We shall often return to this medicine.

9. HARIDRĀ.

The turmeric plant is a tall perennial herb arising from a large ovoid rhizome with cylindrical tubers, orange coloured within.

The rhizome is used in medicine and for cooking. The oblong lanceolate leaves are lily-like and large, they are set in tufts to 1.2 m long. Pale yellow flowers are clustered in dense spikes 10-15 cm long. The plant is native to South East Asia, but it has been introduced to many other areas. It prefers humid conditions and rich loamy soil. Propagation by root division in autumn. Indian (Bengal) turmeric is supposed to be the best. Very common in Indian cooking and as a medicinal plant.

Constituents : volatile oil (5-6%), curcumin (a terpene), starch (24%), albumen (30%). The intense colouring effect is due to curcumin. Turmeric is often used for dying cloth.

—

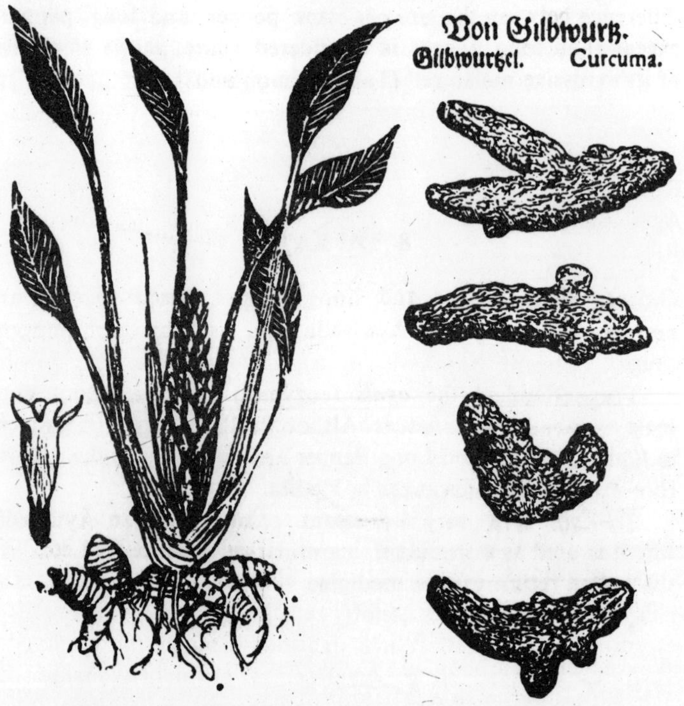

Bot. Name : *Curcuma longa.*
Fam. : Scitaminaceae, Zingiberaceae.
Engl. : Turmeric.

German: Gelbwurtz, Gilbwurtz.

Chinese : *Yu-chin*, *Kiang-hoang* (Mand.) *Keung-hoang* (Cant.).

Rasa : Bitter and pungent.

Vīrya : Hot.

Vipāka : Pungent.

Action : Because it is bitter and pungent (pungent in *vipāka* also): ununctuous, alleviates K and P, only V remains. (Due to its ununctuous nature V is aggravated, for this reason we add a little oil to it). Taken with milk it reduces all three *doṣas*.

Promotes good complexion. As a mask, it clears pimples and cures excessively dry skin. Apply only once at bed-time, leave for two minutes, wash off with luke-warm water, next morning wash off the rest with chick-pea powder (*besun*) and oil, this will remove the yellowish tinge. Take internally as well (corrects liver) in case of acne. Excellent turmeric cream is prepared commercially with sandle wood.

Reduces fat.

Against many skin diseases.

Allergic reaction.

Asthma (fried with a little butter).

Itch of various kinds.

Piles (because it corrects liver blockage. If the liver is not clear, piles may result, if the liver is clear, no piles).

Liver disorders. (Corrects liver, increases bile secretion).

Poisoning from chemicals, insecticides etc.

Chronic rhinitis and sinusitis (closely associated with constipation).

Diabetes (turmeric and *āmalakī* mixed without oil, should be ununctuous to dissolve fat).

Rheumatism, fractures pain due to accidents.

Infections (disinfectant and mild antibiotic).

Intestinal parasites.

Ulcers (turmeric with a little oil).

Cold, cough, fever.

Tubercular adenitis.

Turmeric also reduces cholesterol.

Whether cooked or taken raw, turmeric does not lose its properties.

There is a variety of turmeric which smells like mango fruit, this is known as *Āmba-Haridrā* (*Curcuma amada*), wrestlers use this against pains and sprains.

Use in Chinese medicine : Stimulates energy circulation and relieves congestion. "cools the blood", dispels the troubles of "black blood". Used against rheumatic pain, heart and stomach pains, amenorrhea, formation of pus. Acts upon the spleen meridian. Considered to be of cold properties and acrid to taste.

Use in Western medicine : Warm and dry in nature, aromatic and stimulant. Against impure blood, catarrh, purulent ophthalmia, good for cold and weak stomach, tonifies liver and spleen, also used against long term disorders of these organs.

10. LASUNA

Garlic is a perennial or biennial plant widely cultivated as a vegetable. The best varieties grow in warm climate.

The bulbs have about 8-20 cloves surrounded by silky whitish skin. Flat, erect, long pointed leaves about 15 cm long and 1—2.5 cm wide, arise from the base.

The stem upto 10 cm long is unbranched and bears apical small dense umbels of rose-white to greenish flowers.

Garlic is a native of Asia, today it is cultivated in many countries of the world. Prefers rich, light well drained soils. Individual cloves are planted 4 cm deep and 15 cm apart for cultivation.

Constituents : Essential oil, comprising mainly allyl disulphide and allyl propyl disulphide; vitamins A, B1, B2 and C; anti-bacterial substances comprising allicin, allicetoin I and II; also an enzyme allinase.

There is a variety of garlic with only one clove called *Eka Kalī Lasuna*.

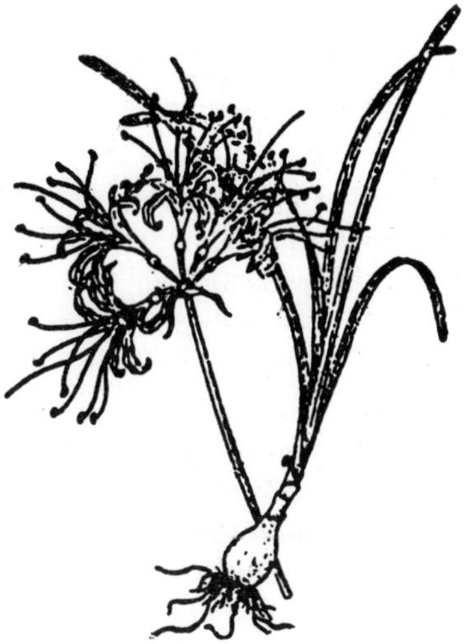

Bot. Name : *Allium sativum*

Fam. : Liliaceae.

Engl. : Garlic.

German : Knoblauch.

Chinese : Shih-Suan, Hsiao Suan, Suan.

Arabic : Chaum.

Greek : Σ/<όγοδ√

Rasa : Sweet, saline, pungent; bitter astringent (no sour taste).

Vīrya : Hot. (Good for V-K disease, for paitiko constitution patients, give less).

Vipāka :

Action : Strengthens voice, complexion, intellect, eye—sight, memory.
Nourishment.
Rejuvenation.
Digestive.
Gives Longevity.
Pain killer.
Haemopoetic.
Cardiac tonic.

Good for hair and sterility.

Used against : Various types of skin diseases.
Phantom tumors.
Infections.
Piles.
Colic pains.
Chronic fever.
Anorexia.
Bronchitis.
Heart diseases.
Urinary disorders.
Rheumatism.
Sinusitis.
Epilepsy.

Garlic is used in rejuvenation therapy, which should be carried out during the winter. Physical constitution should be strong for this treatment, and the body and mind of the patient should be prepared to accept the treatment, which implies 15 g of garlic per day as least. Complications may include vomiting and fainting.

A very suitable vehicle to administrate garlic is alcohol or wine.

Use in Chinese medicine : Warm and acrid to taste, detoxifies, reduces swelling anthelmintic. Warms central organs and opens stoppages, cleanses intestines. Diarrhoea and dysentery, colds, blocked nose, tuberculosis (with cough), ringworm, boils, abscesses.

Use in Western medicine : Warm and dry in the fourth degree. Penetrates, thins. Antibacterial, hypotensive, expectorant, anthelmintic, fungicide, carminative, protects against common cold, increases bile fluid. According to Tabernaemontanus garlic is at its best in the second month after planting. After harvesting it should be hung up to keep its properties upto one year. It warms and dries a cold stomach, breaks up thick moisture, opens channels, carminative, detoxifies, rejuvenates, gives good voice. Also used against kidney stones.

Calcined garlic (*bhasma*) with honey is used externally against various skin disorders.

11. BRĀHMĪ

Two species are known as *Brāhmī* in āyurvedic medicine.

1. *Hydrocotyle asiatica* or Indian Pennywort, is a slender, trailing umbelliferous plant with reddish prostrate stems rooting at the nodes. Petioles to 15 cm tall bear glabrous somewhat reniform leaves 1-15 cm long. Flowerheads bear 3 or 6 reddish flowers.

Costituents : A heteroside (saponoside), asiaticoside (which is antibiotic) and also assists in the formation of scar tissue; triterpene acids; a glycoside, indocentellocide; an alkaloid, hydrocotylin; resin; pectic acid; vitamin C; a bitter compound, vellarin; tannin (9%); sugars; volatile oil.

Bot. Name : *Hydrocotyle asiatica*

Fam : Umbelliferae.

Engl. : Indian Pennywort.

German : Asiatischer Wassernabel.

Chinese : *Man-t'ien-hsing.* It is often called *Fo-ti-tieng.* Many writers claim that *Fo-ti-tieng* is the name of this herb, but according to Dr. P. Airola, *Fo-ti-tieng* is a trade name for a herbal formula made from three different herbs one of which is *Hydrocotyle asiatica* Minor.

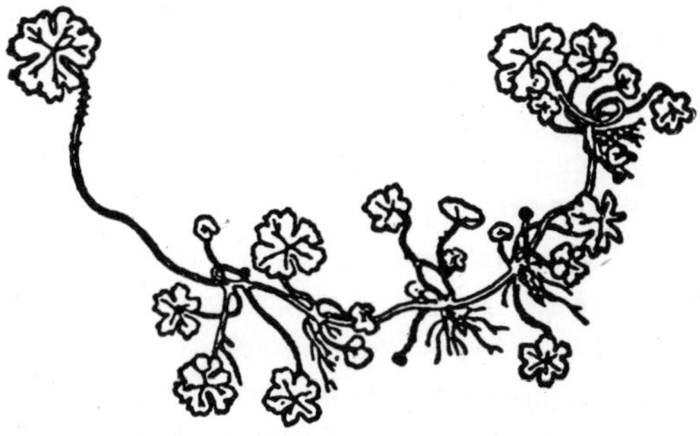

2. *Bacopa Monnieri* (earlier name : *Herpestris Monnieri*) This species grows near water in sandy places.

Fam. : Scrophulaceae

The first mentioned species is more used for the voice, the second species more for good memory, otherwise their action is very similar. In both cases :

Rasa : Bitter, pungent and sweet.

Vīrya : Cold (good for the nervous system. Any drug which has a soothing effect on the nerves is cold in potency. Useful in many P conditions).

Vipāka : Sweet.

Action : Promotes longevity.
Good memory and sleep.
Good voice and complexion.
Rejuvenating.
Used against : Fever and skin diseases (bitter, therefore blood purifier).
Cough (asthma), bronchitis. (Indirect action, but because of cold nature not very effective).
Bleeding (cooling).
Heart diseases.
Diabetes.
Adenitis.

Brāhmī Rasāyana is a tonic jam.

Brāhmī boiled in sesame oil (*Brāhmī Taila*) is wonderful before sleep. (The sesame oil is heating, but it becomes cool in character when boiled with *Brāhmī* or *Āmalakī*. The oil takes the effect of the plant).

Brāhmī powder with gold and pearl as a pill is used against nervous exhaustion and epilepsy.

In case of P aggravation add a little water to the preparations with sesame oil, to further reduce the hot character of the oil.

Hydrocotyle Asiatica in Chinese medicine : Cooling, pleasant to taste but slightly acrid. Clears fever and detoxifies, resolves mucus. Colds and flu, cough, sore throat, boils and abscesses, jaundice, liver, cirrhosis.

Hydrocotyle Asiatica in Western medicine : Tonic, diuretic, purgative.

Bacopa Monniera in Chinese medicine : Slightly warm, pleasant and somewhat biting to taste. Warms kidneys and stimulates *Yang* energy. Used for impotence, premature ejaculation, back aches, cold uterus, irregular menstruation' rheumatism.

Chinese Name ; *Pa-chi-t'ien.*

12. VACĀ

Sweet Flag, also called Sweet Sedge, Myrtle Flag or Calmus, is a hardy vigorous, aromatic perennial. The branched rhizome, about 3 cm thick, bears sword shaped leaves with wavy margins, upto 1 m high and about 15 cm wide.

Ackerwurtz. Acorum.

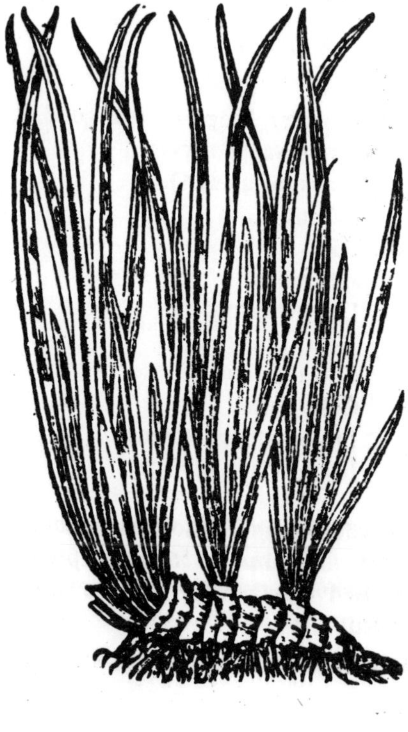

In early summer an inflorescence of about 4-8 cm length bears small flowers.

Calmus is indigenous to Central Asia and Eastern Europe. Now it is found in many parts of the world in marshy regions. It needs moist soil and frequent watering, grows best by water margins. Calmus is found from the equator to the snow line, in tropical climate as well as in high altitudes.

Constituents: Bitter aromatic volatile oil; bitter principle called acorin.

Bot. Name : *Acorus calamus.*
Fam. : Araceae,
Engl. : Sweet Flag, Sweet Sedge, Myrtle Flag, Calmus.
German: Ackerwurtz, Kalmus.
Chinese: Ch'ang-p'u
Greek: α/<oὸos, α/<oδor.
Arabic: Vage.
Rasa: Pungent, bitter.
Vīrya: Hot (wheras *Brāhmī* is cold).
Vipāka: Pungent.

Action: Promotes memory, longevity and good voice.
Emetic (acts on vagus nerve).
Liberates sinus (as a snuff).
Alleviates V and K.
Against: Piles.
Infections.
Uterine disorders.
Heart diseases.
Constipation.
Colic pains.
Distension of stomach.
Insanity and epilepsy.

Vacā is more effective in V disorders (mental) than *Brāhmī*. If P is aggravated, use *Brāhmī*. In many preparations *Brāhmī* and *Vacā* are used together, for instance to *Brāhmī Rasāyana Vacā* is also added.

Vacā is also used in fumigations against evil spirits traditionally.

Use in Chinese medicine: Neutral in nature, biting to taste, expels gas, alleviates constipation, resolves phlegm, kills worms and detoxifies.

Used against epilepsy and strokes, rheumatoid arthritis, stomach ache, edema, toxic dysentery.

Use in Western medicine: Warm and dry in the third degree, subtle in substance, divides and breaks up, opener and cleanser.

Carminative, vermifuge, spasmolytic, diaphoretic, diuretic. Stimulates salivary and gastric glands, slight sedative action on central nervous system. Against flatulent colic, dyspepsia. Against hardened spleen, stomach, cramps cold liver and spleen.

13. TULSĪ

Sacred Basil, a relative of Sweet Basil, is a variety of Basil much used in āyurvedic medicine. The plant enjoys a sacred status in India. In Australia *Tulasī* grows in Queensland and the Northern Territory.

The species is rarely described in Western texts of botanic medicine, but Tabernaemontanus describes it as having bluish, crisp, serrated leaves, and as being of very beautiful fragrance. In ancient Italian texts the species is sometimes mentioned as *Ocimum Crispum Hispanicum*.

The stem is about 40 cm high, a little rough and often brownish red. The smooth leaves are about 2.5 cm broad and roundish, sometimes blackish reddish, sometimes bluish. The flower is white-red. In India *Tulasī* is found in many home gardens.

Bot. Name: *Ocimum Sanctum*.

Fam.: Labiatae.

Engl: Sacred Basil, Black Basil.

German: Breit-krauses Basilikum.

The plant is an annual, but by not allowing it to form seeds, it becomes practically a perennial.

Rasa : Bitter, pungent and astringent.

Vīrya : Hot.

Vipāka : Sweet.

Action : *Tulasī* contains copper in organic ionized form. Regular intake of this plant increases immunity. *Tulasī* has a good effect on the mind (tranquility, mental peace). It is commonly used in herb teas, also with milk and sugar.

Tulasi makes the body light and avoids accumulation of fat, specially in ladies after the menopause.

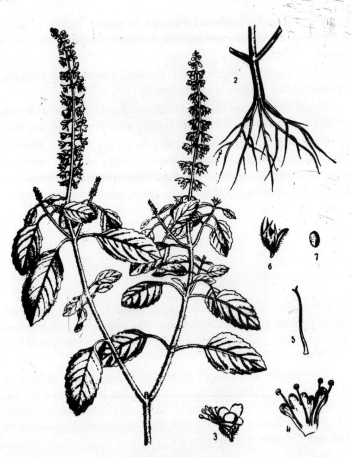

Breit krauſe Baſilien.

IV. Ocimum latifolium criſpum. C. B.

It reduces K but alleviates all three *doṣas*.

As a tea it is taken as one teaspoon of powder or leaves per cup, twice daily in case of adults. Also taken in honey, which reinforces its action (a quarter teaspoon in honey).

Useful for gastro-intestinal tract and lungs, liver disorders (not powerful stimulant for adults).

Copper contains a lot of *agni mahābhūta*.

Use in Western medicine: Warm in the second degree. Expectorant, strengthens heart, against depression, as a tonic, galactogogue, aphrodisiac.

14. YAṢṬIMADHU

Liquorice has been used medically for thousands of years. The herbaceous perennial 0.5 to 1.5 cm tall, has a tap root of

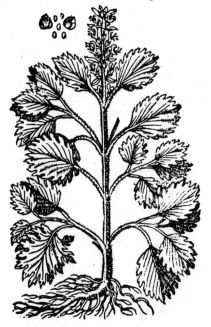

about 15 cm length which subdivides into 3-5 subsidiary roots 1.25 cm in length and several horizontal stolons which may reach 8 m. The erect stem bears 4-7 pairs of leaflets, 2.5-5 cm long, ovate, glutinous underneath. 1 cm long flowers, lilac blue, in loose racemes 10-15 cm long, appear in mid or late summer, followed by reddish brown pods 1-2.5 cm long. Grows well on deep sandy soils, often in river valleys. Propagated by root division.

Constituents : Glycyrrhizin (5-10%), comprising calcium and potassium salts of glycyrrhizic acid; flavonoid glycosides, liquiritoside, isoliquiritoside; sucrose and dextrose (5-10%); starch (30%); protein, fat; resin; asparagin; volatile oil; saponins. Liquorice is widely used in medicine, it is also part of the British and U.S., pharmacopoeia, but its use in

Glycyrrhiza.

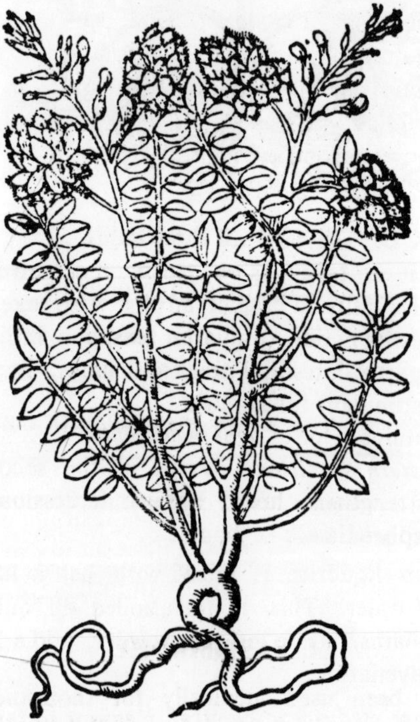

modern medicine is limited as an expectorant. The plant does not grow in India, since recently however, it is being cultivated on Indian soil.

Bot. Name : *Glycyrrhiza glabra*
Fam. : Leguminosae
Engl. : Liquorice
German : Süßholz, Süßholzwurzel
Chinese : Ling-t'ung, luo-laor, lu ts'ao, mei-ts'ao, mi-kan, mi-ts'ao.
Rasa : Sweet
Vīrya : Cold
Vipāka : Sweet
Since its potency is cold and its *vipāka* sweet, it would normally not act on K. But it actually liquifies and alleviates K. Its action is anabolic. Used for P and V alleviation as well.
Action : promotes longevity and healing powers
strengthens in case of fatigue
Laxative (enema), to eliminate V
Emetic (smooth painless vomiting)
Tonic
Promotes good eyesight
Against : rheumatism
bleeding (but not as powerful as *Vāsā*, see, no. 15)
throat irritation, bronchitis
urinary disorders
morbid thirst
exhaustion
Alleviates P, V and K (expectorant), removes K from the body.

Mostly used in powder form. The root is fibrous, it is therefore boiled, mixed with milk or honey.

1 tablespoon liquorice is mixed with half a litre of milk and two litres of water. This is then boiled till only half a litre of liquid remains. Strain off the powder, add a little sugar and give for rejuvenation.

Use in Chinese medicine: : Neutral, pleasant to taste, Revitalizes the centre and supplements energy, detoxifies and loosens phlegm. Mediates between the medicines it is combined with.

Use in Western medicine : Of temperate nature almost equal to the warmth of humans. Expectorant, demulcent, laxative, spasmolytic, anti-inflammatory.

15. VĀSĀ

The Malabar Nut Tree is actually a bush about 2 m high. The leaves are 8-15 cm long, about 5 cm wide, lanceolate, of dull brownish colour when dried. The taste is bitter, the smell like that of strong tea. The beautiful flower has the shape of a lion's mouth. Its wood is soft and makes excellent coal for gunpowder.

Constituents : The leaves contain a bitter crystalline alkaloid Vasicine, and an organic adhatodic acid, another alkaloid and an odourous volatile principle. The whole plant is used in medicine.

Bot. Name : *Adhatoda vasica*
Fam. : Acanthaceae.
Engl. : Malabar Nut Tree.
Rasa : Bitter.
Vīrya : Cold.
Vipāka : Pungent.
Action : Alleviates K and P.
Against : all kinds of bleeding
bronchitis (expectorant). For chronic cough a jam is prepared by adding sugar. This is also good against constipation. Since *Vāsā* is bitter and cold, it regulates P and is therefore good for liver-fever and asthma.
Jaundice.
Fever.
Asthma (often smoked along with *Dhaturā* leaves).

Adhatoda vasica nees

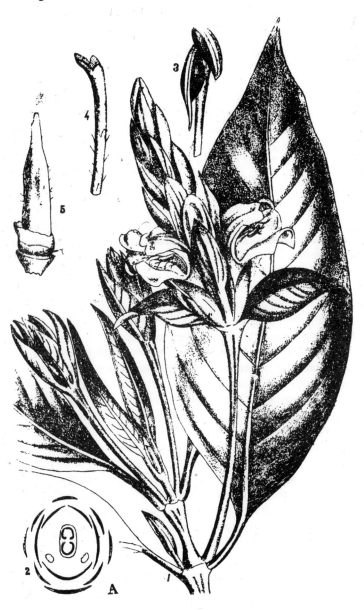

Skin diseases (taken internally and applied externally).
Tuberculosis.
Kidney diseases (acts as a diurctic).
Ulcers.
Wounds.
Conjunctivitis (juice of flower).

Vāsāyām vidyamānāyām
aśāyām jīvitasya ca
raktapitti kṣayi kuṣṭnı
kimartham avasīdasi.

(Since there is a drug called *Vāsā* in existence which is the hope of life, bleeding from different parts of the body, diminished one, suffering from obstinate skin disease, with what motive are you sorrowful?)

16. JĀTIPHALA

Nutmeg is a tall, bushy evergreen tree which grows to about 12 m. The leaves are yellowish, eliptic or lanceolate, about 5-12 cm long. Flowers in axillary umbels are 6mm long, they are followed by a nearly globular or pear shaped red or yellow fruit, which splits to release the ovoid seed surrounded by a scarlet outer covering. The seed is known as nutmeg, the outer covering as mace.

The tree is native to the Molucca Islands, now widespread in the tropics. Trees produce fruits in the 9th or 10th year and may last for 80 years. Propagated from cuttings.

Constituents : (kernel) volatile oil (5-15%); fixed oil (25-40%) comprising myristic acid (60%), oleic, palmitic, lauric and lionoleic acid; also terpineol, borneol and terpenes.

Bot. Name : *Myristica fragrans.*
Fam : Myristicaceae.
Engl. : Nutmeg.
German : Muskatbaum.
Rasa : Pungent, bitter, astringent.
Vīrya : Hot.

Nux muſchata.

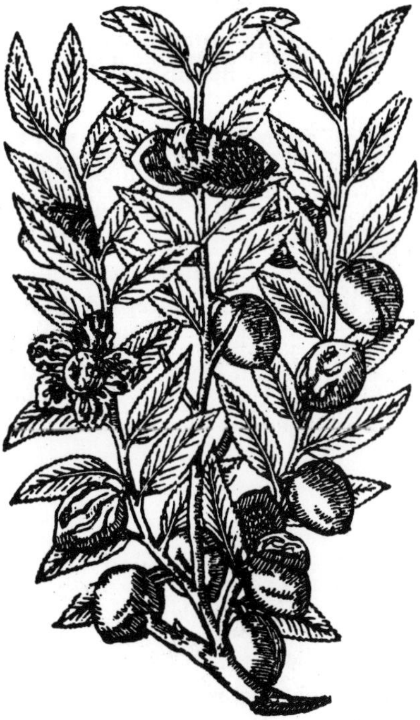

Vipāka : Pungent.
Action : Stimulates digestion.

Constipative but *anulomana,* stops diarrhoea, no stomach distension.

Alleviates K and V.

Good for voice.

Against : stickness in the mouth and bad breath,
throat disease,
urinary disorders,
fever,
cough,
vomiting,
āsthmā,
heart diseases,

pain in abdomen,
uterine disorders.

Nutmeg is considered an aphrodisiac, it increases the power of retention of semen. Because of its narcotic effect it induces sleep.

If given to ladies after delivery there will be no uterine problems, no sepsis etc. Useful for children when rubbed and mixed with honey or milk, for good sleep and teething trouble, and to avoid digestive trouble.

Use in Western medicine : Carminative, aromatic, stimulant. Used in small doses to reduce flatulence, aid digestion, improve the appetite and to treat diarrhoea, vomiting and nausea. To be used sparingly, overdose can cause disorientation, hallucinations and convulsions. Tabernaemontanus describes nutmeg as warm in the second degree and astringent.

17. HIṄGU

Hiṅgu (Asafoetida) is a strongly foetid brownish resinous latex which comes from a perennial plant, which grows upto more than 2 m hight, having large bipinnate radical leaves and developing a massive fleshy rootstock. The inflorescence is produced in the 5th year of growth on a thick flowering stem to 10 cm thick and to 3 m high. Yellow flowers in umbels appear in mid-spring. Native to Eastern Persia and Western Afghanistan. From Afghanistan it is imported into India as Milk of Asafoetida. This is the dried gum, unfortunately it is often adulterated. Actually two species serve as the source of Asafoetida, 1. Ferula narthex Boiss, 2. Ferula foetida Regel. The plants look almost identical. The resinous gum is collected from plants which are at least five years old. Constituents: volatile oil (10%); resin (50%); gum (25%) ferulic acid. The volatile oil contains terpenes, disulphides and pinene, and is mainly responsible for the therapeutic action of the species.

Bot. Name: *Ferula narthex* / *Ferula foetida* } Both species almost look identical.

* Ferulkraut. Ferula. *

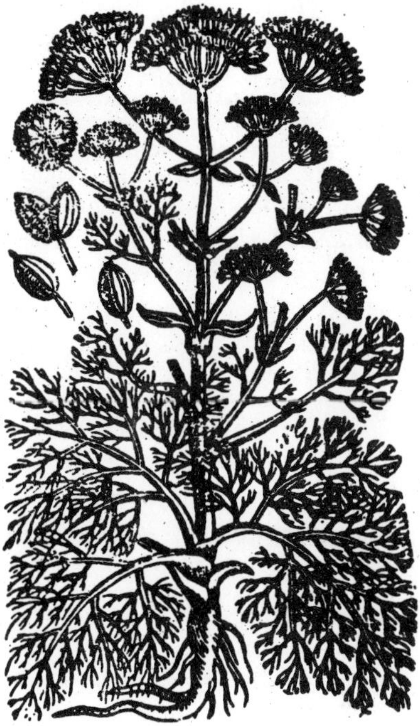

Fam.: Umbelliferae.

Engl.: Asafoetida, "Devil's Dung".

German: Asafoetida, Teufelsdreck.

Rasa: Pungent
Vīrya: Hot
) for this reason a digestive stimulant, stimulates *agnis* in digestive tract and tissues.

Vipāka: Pungent.

Action: Digestive stimulant.

Carminative.

Alleviates V and K. (Because of its hot property it is not so useful for patients with P constitution or with P aggravation).

Stimulates nerves.
Expectorant.
Diuretic.
Emmenagogue (misused for abortion).
Against: Intestinal perasites (creates a hostile atmosphere).
Constipation (helps downward movement of wind).
Colic pain (stimulates liver, bile secretion).
Whooping cough.
Paralysis.
Sciatica.

For Heat Pain, Pneumonia: *Hingu* 1 pt
Camphor 1 pt
Musk 1/8th pt
Make pills of 250 mg. Take 1 pill with hot water.

Hingu fried in a little butter will become crisp. Keep for use, it counteracts the bad smell of garlic.

Use in Western medicine: Nervine stimulant, powerful antispasmodic, expectorant, carminative. Very effective in hysteria, bronchitis, asthma and whooping cough, flatulent colic. According to Tabernaemontanus it also warms and dries, and its *bhasma* stops bleeding.

18. GUGGULU

Myrrha or Gum Myrrh is a low bush or small tree to 2.75 m high. The trunk is thick and bears numerous irregular, knotted branches and smaller clustered branchlets which spread at right angles and terminate in a spine. Few leaves about 1-1.5 cm long at the end of short branchlets, trifoliate with minute lateral leaflets, the terminal 1 cm long, of obovate-oval shape. The leaves are glabrous. A gum is discharged through the bark naturally or after wounding. The species loves basaltic

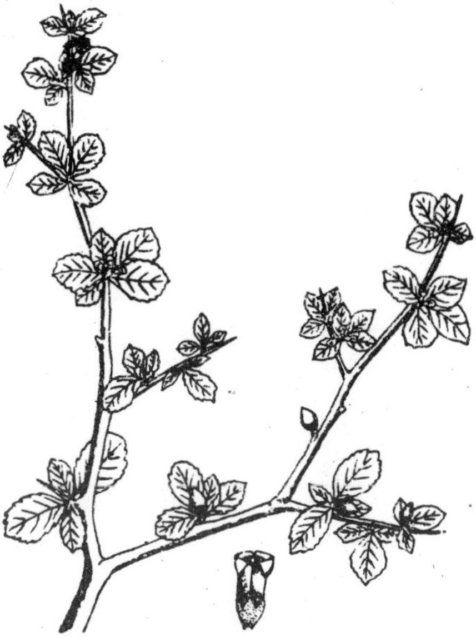

land in very hot areas. Constituents: Oleo-gum-resin, comprising 25-35% resin, 2.5—6.5% volatile oil, 50-60% gum.

The plant has pink-red flowers in spring, fruit in summer. It is propagated by cuttings. The plant needs very little water for growth. The resin, which is also used in incense, is collected after cutting the stem.

Bot. Name: *Commiphora mukul.*

Fam. Burseraceae.

Engl.: Myrrh.

German: Myrrhe.

Chinese: Mo-yao.

Greek: μυϱῖ́γη.

Rasa: Pungent.

Vīrya: Hot.

Vipāka: Pungent.

Action: *Guggulu* has strong power to alleviate K and *āma*, it also reduces fat. Since it is an *oily* resin, it also alleviates V.

Rejuvenation.

Cardiac tonic.
Heals: fractures.
ulcers.
pain in joints.
urinary disorders.
edema,
adiposity.
hyper cholesterolemia.
lymphadenitis (enlargement of lymphglands and their inflammation).
goitre (acts on swelling and hormones—pituitary gland).
skin diseases.
parasites.
is nourishing as well as depleting (balances the situation).

Use in Chinese medicine: Neutral, bitter to taste. Reduces swelling and localizes pain. For traumatic injuries and pain, carbuncles and sores, pains in the chest and abdominal region, rheumatism, amenorrhea and dysmenorrhea.

Use in Western medicine: Of medium nature as far as cold and warm is concerned, drying, astringent. The berries as a cardiac tonic. Leaves against boils, bad body odour, abscesses in the mouth, astringent to mucous membranes, tincture for ulcers, constituent of some tooth powders. In veterinary medicine for wound treatment, used in incense.

19. JIRAKA

Cumin is a slender, glabrous annual herb about 15 cm high; branched stems above: leaves with filiform divisions 15 mm—5 cm long; sparsely flowered umbels, white or rose coloured appear in late spring. The bristly fruit is 7 mm long.

Constituents: Essential oil, 2.5-4% comprising cumaldehyde, terpenes, cuminic alcohol, pinenes; also fatty oil and pentosan. The dried ripe fruit is used.

For cultivation seeds are sown in late spring in sandy soil in a warm situation, plants are thinned out to 20 cm apart. Cultivated on the North African coast, Middle East, India, Malta and China.

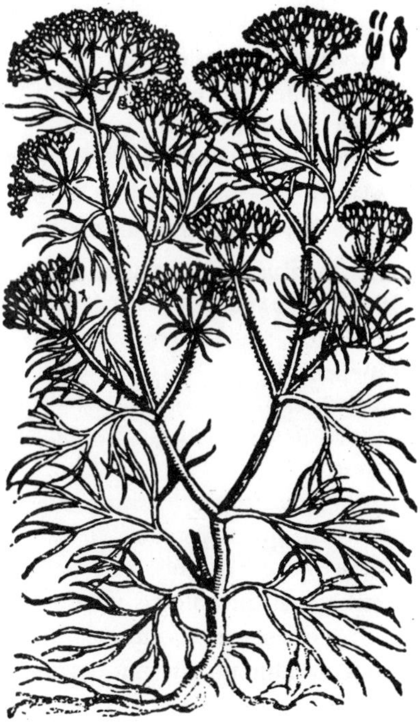

Bot. Name: *Cuminum cyminum* L.
Fam.: Umbelliferae.
Engl.: Cumin,
German: Pfefferkümmel.
Rasa Pungent.
Vīrya: Hot.
Vipāka: Pungent.
The black variety has the botanical name: *Carum Carvi* (Engl. Caraway), from the ancient Arabic : Karawiya. German: Kümmel.
Action: Digestive.
Stimulant.

Carminative.
Alleviates K and V.
Against: Colic pains,
phantom tumors,
diarrhoea,
sprue syndrome,
chronic states of fever,
vomiting,
piles.
Split a ripe banana and fill it with cumin seed or powder, take this for good sleep.

The powder is often given to ladies after delivery.

Use in Western medicine: Warming, thinning, digestive, divides, opens, dries and expells. Warm in the third and dry in the early part of the third degree. Digestive, carminative, diarrhoea and dyspepsia.

20. TILA

Sesame is widely cultivated for its oil. The plant is an erect, strongly smelling, finely pubescent annual, 90 cm tall. Variable leaves (lanceolate or oblong, alternate or opposite). Flowers are purple to whitish, 3 cm long, followed by a 3 cm long capsule containing numerous flat seeds. There are several varieties, a black and a white variety. Sometimes the black seed is also made white by removing the husk, but this is different. The plant is a native of the tropics. Constituents: fixed oil (55%), a phenolic substance, sesamal, sesamin, choline; lecithin; nicotinic acid; calcium salts.

Bot. Name: *Sesamum indicum*.
Fam.: Pedaliaceae.
Engl.: Sesame, Benne, Gingilly, Teel.
German: Leindotter.
Chinese: *Hei Chih-ma*.
Greek: Σηδαμοr.
Rasa: Sweet, Pungent.

Leindotter. Sesamum.

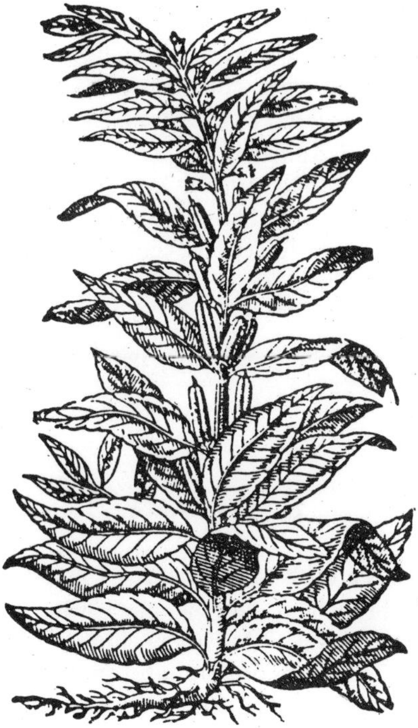

Vīrya: Hot.
Vipāka: Sweet
Action: Alleviates *vāyu* (the best for alleviating V).
Stimulates digestion.
Promotes memory.
Rejuvenating.
Good for eye sight.
Used for: Adiposity.
Uterine disorders (emmenagogue).
Urinary disorders.
Injuries.

If medicines are boiled in sesame oil, the oil captures the medicine and becomes its carrier, (*Saṁskārāt guṇa kāraka*). It

is *yogavāha*, i.e. it enhances or strengthens the medicines which are added to it.

Use in Chinese medicine: Neutral, pleasant to taste. Strengthens liver and kidneys, moistens the five viscera (*chuang*). Against inadequate liver and kidney function, head-cold, dizziness, numbness and paralysis, constipation. Chases *Fong* (wind), against excessive dryness, general tonic, acts on meridians of liver, colon, lung and kidneys.

Use in Western medicine: Has a fat oily moisture, slightly warm, softens, pacifies. Nutritive laxative, emollient, demulcent, for genito-urinary, infections, constipation, ground seeds with water against haemorrhoids, good emmenagogue.

21. VĀTĀMA

The almond tree is a bush or tree from 3-7 m tall, with glabrous light coloured branches, narrow glabrous, finely dentate, oblong-lanceolate leaves 7.5—10 cm long, with gland bearing petiole. Usually solitary flowers are pink or white, 3-4 cm wide, from mid to late spring, followed by oblong-ovoid light green pubescent fruits 4 cm long, containing, 2 seeds.

Native to southern and Central Asia, specially Persia. Grows upto 3000 m altitude. Seed constituents: protein (20%); fatty oil (65%), enzymes, mainly emulsin; vitamins A, Bl, B2, B, B6, E and PP (nicotinamide): mineral salts. Bitter almonds contain upto 4% of a toxic glycoside (amygdalin). Raw bitter almonds are poisonous, they contain cyanide derivatives. The almond tree is widely cultivated in many parts of the world.

Bot. Name: ***Prunus amygdalus, Amygdalus communis.***
Fam.: Rosaceae.
Engl: Almond tree.
German: Mandelbaum.
Chinese: Hsieng-jen.

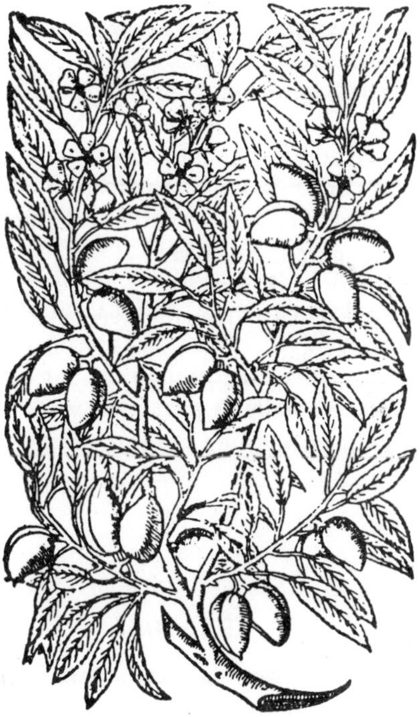

Greek: αμυγδαλη

Rasa: Sweet, Pungent, Bitter.

Vīrya: Hot.

Vipāka: Sweet.

Action: Alleviates V.
- Nourishing.
- Strength promoting.
- For:
  - Lung diseases.
  - Kidney diseases.
  - Pain in the back: make a paste from almonds, cloves, cardamom, cinnamon + a little black pepper.
  - Excellent nervine tonic: 1 spoon of almond oil every morning or evening in milk (which has cooling effect) gives good sleep.

Aphrodisiac recipe: Almond + *Aśvagandhā* (*Withania somnifera*) + *Pippalī* + Ghee + Milk + Sugar. Take for 1 month. Also gives good sleep.

Inhalation of almond oil soothes nerves (goes to sinus and a part gets absorbed by nerve tissue, good effect on brain).

Use in Chinese medicine: Warming properties, acrid but pleasant to taste. Resolves phlegm and quiets cough, lowers excessive energy, lubricates intestines. Good for colds, cough, unproductive coughing, dyspnoea, asthma, constipation.

Use in Western medicine: Warm and dry or warm and moist. Demulcent, nutritive. For cough mixtures, the oil is much used as massage oil and internally as a laxative, while the whole seed is slightly constipating according to some ancient authors.

22. ERAṆḌA

The Castor Oil plant is a very variable annual herb or perennial tree from 2-15 m tall, usually about 4 m. Leaves are simple, alternate, with 5-11 lobes, on long petioles, glossy, upto 1m wide. Flowers are male below, female above, both without petals and in panicles, are followed by a smooth or spiny capsule, 3 cm in diameter. Native to India and tropical Africa. Grows throughout tropical and many temperate regions. Loves well drained soil and full sun. Cultivated commercially in many countries. Propagated from seed planted in early spring. Constituents: (seed) protein (26%); fixed oil (50%) comprising ricinoleic, oleic, linoleic, stearic and hydroxy stearic acids. One of the protein substances in the whole seed is a toxic albuminoid, to which a poisonous effect is due. There are several varieties of this plant. Mainly the seeds of this plant are given, but the leaves, root and stem are also useful.

Bot. Name: *Ricinus communis*.
Fam: Euphorbiaceae.
Engl.: Castor Oil plant.
German: Ricinus Baum.

Chinese: P' i-ma.
Greek: *kíkι, πενταδα'κτυλος*
Rasa: Pungent, Bitter, Sweet.
Vīrya: Hot.
Vipāka: Pungent.

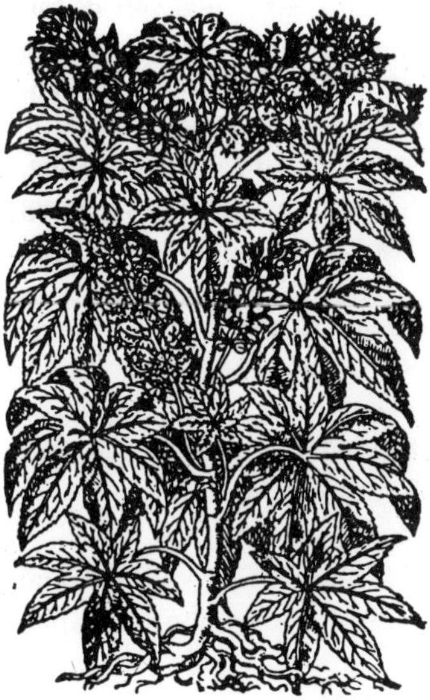

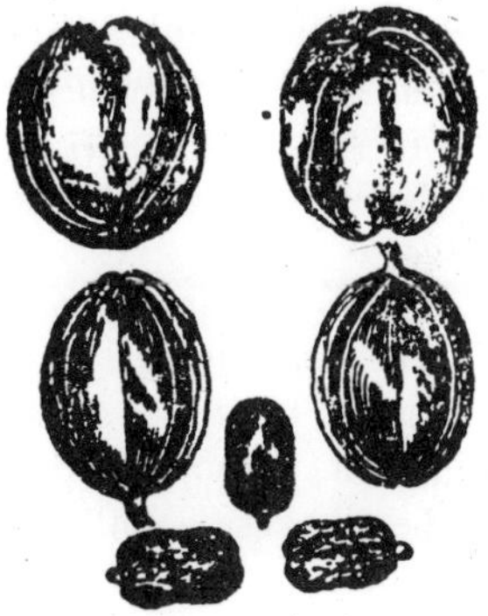

Action : The oil is good for all rheumatic diseases. Given raw, it acts as a purgative. The refined oil is much less effective.

Useful in cases of : Gout.
Rheumatoid arthritis.
Asthma.
Bronchitis.
Stones.
Phantom tumors.
Colic pain.
Early stages of appendicitis. (Operation can be avoided, since the oil works as an emollient over an inflamed appendix, but it has to be kept in mind that it acts as a strong purgative, therefore only 1/8 of a spoon is added to some sweet).

A bandage of the leaves of this plant, made warm, can be applied to joints or other parts of the body which pains. Sometimes the leaves are combined with leaves of *Dhaturā*. A massage with warm castor oil is good for pain. Since the oil is somewhat greasy, a hot bath is taken afterwards, add some decoction of leaves to the bath-water. The root and stem can be used in fomentation.

Use in Chinese medicine: Nautral, pleasant to taste, but slightly acrid and slightly toxic. Draws out pus, stops pain, relieves constipation, corrects prolapses. For wounds, boils and abscesses, enlarged lymph nodes, joint pains, strabismus and facial palsy, constipation, anal and uterine prolapse.

Use in Western medicine : Principally as a purgative in case of chronic constipation. Applied as an enema to remove impacted feaces, externally as an emollient. Soothing to eye irritation. Whole seeds are considered toxic and large doses of the oil cause vomiting, colic and severe purgation.

23. VATSANĀBHA

Three species of Aconite go under this name. All the species contain an active poison. Aconitine is present in all parts of the plant, but specially in the root. Aconitine is more poisonous than prussic acid and acts with tremendous rapidity. One fiftieth grain kills a sparrow in a few seconds, one tenth a rabbit in five minutes.

Aconitum ferox is the most powerful of the species. Poisoning of wells by this plant has been carried out in India in order to stop an advancing army. The name Aconite derives from the Greek *akontion* meaning a dart, it was obviously used to poison arrows. The species known as *Aconitum chasmanthum* contains Indaconitine, while the type *Aconitum palmatum* yield an alkaloid called Palmatisine.

The species are hardy perennials. During the first year the root is produced, during the second year the flowering stem, about 1.5 m high, with dark green, glossy divided leaves about 3-8 cm wide. In summer and autumn violet-blue flowers are produced in terminal clusters, the flowers are helmet shaped. Prefers moist soils. Propagation by root division in autumn.

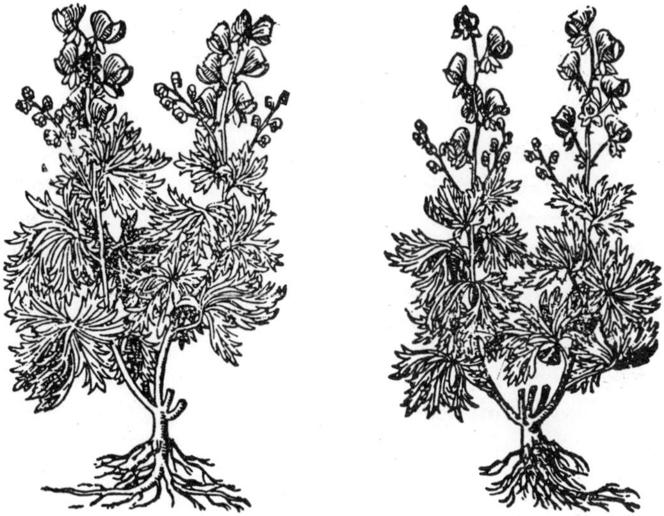

Bot. Name : *Aconitum ferox,*
Accnitum chasmanthum,
Aconitum palmatum.

Fam. : Ranunculaceae.

Engl. : Aconite, Monk's Hood, Blue Rocket, Friar's Cap.

German : Blauer Eisenhut, Sturmhut.

Chinese : (*Aconitum lycotonum*) Ch'uan wu.

Rasa : Sweet, Pungent.

Vīrya : Hot.

Vipāka : Pungent.

Action : Alleviates K and V.

Used against : Skin diseases.
Edema.
Asthma.
Bronchitis.
Ascitis.
Fever (*sannipāta* type).

Diabetes mellitus.
Ext. Ulcers.
Cervical Lymphadenitis.
Internal swelling.

The plant has to be purified (made non-poisonous) with cow's milk. It is cut into pieces and soaked in milk for 7 days after removing the outer bark. It is then washed in cold water. This process has to be repeated, sometimes 2-3 times, till the taste does not produce any numbness on the tongue.

Use in Chinese medicine : (*Aconitum lycotonum*) slightly warm, biting to taste, extremely toxic. Eliminates cold caused by moisture, opens up meridian passage ways, alleviates cold caused aches and pains. Against wind and cold caused moisture numbness, wind caused joint pains, spasms of extremities, windblown headache, chest and abdominal pain.

Use in Western medicine: Sedative; pain killer; antipyretic. Externally for neuralgia and sciatica. Of great importance in Homoeopathic medicine.

24. ATIVIṢĀ

Atikrānta=which overcomes, *viṣā*=poison, the name indicates therefore : the plant which can overcome poisonous effects. Actually this is a non-poisonous form of Aconite, "that which has overcome poisonous nature." The plant does not contain Aconitine. Its chief constituent is an intensely bitter alkaloid called Atisine, possessing tonic and anti-periodic principles.

Bot. Name : *Aconitum heterophyllum.*
Fam. : Ranunculaceae.
Rasa : Bitter, Sweet.
Vīrya : Hot.
Vipāka : Sweet.
Action : Alleviates V, P, K.
Digestive stimulant.

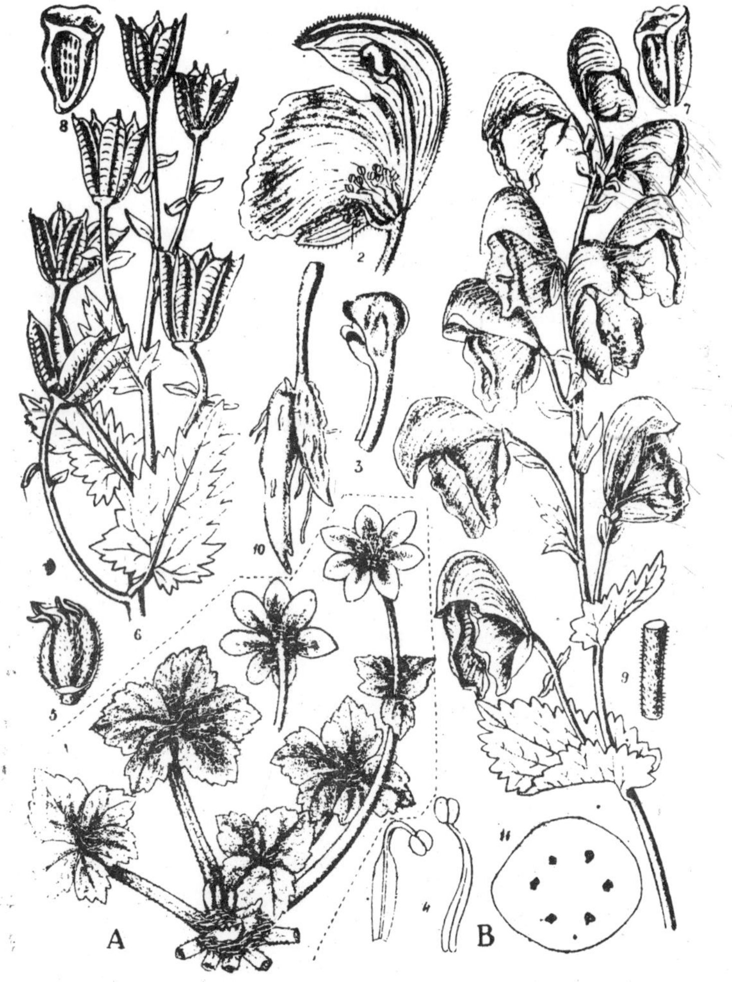

Aconitum Hete rophyllum wall

Tonic.

Carminative.

Purifies mother's milk. (After delivery the milk of mothers may be polluted and affected by V, K or P. Because of this *doṣa*, pollution the milk may not be suitable for the child. With this plant the milk can be purifie d).

Used against : Malaise.
Diarrhoea.
Sprue syndrome.
Cough, Cold.
Vomiting, Colic pain.
Dysentery.
Bleeding, Piles.

The plant is non-poisonous and can even be given to a small child. Good preventive also.

25. VIḌANGA

Shrub or tree about 3.5 to 4.5 m high, which grows in cold places in high altitudes. Petiolate leaves and small, whity pink flowers in racemes at the end of branches. The berries are small spherical fruits, resembling pepper corns, they vary in colour from red to black. The fruits of *Embelia ribes* have ovate, lanceolate smooth leaves and warty fruits and sometimes used to adulterate pepper. The fruits of *Embelia robusta* are longitudinally finely striated. Constituents : Embelic acid (soluble only in alcohol, chloroform or benzem) and a quinone called *Embelia.*

Bot. Name: *Embelia ribes.*
Fam.: Myrsinaceae.
Engl.: Embelia, Viranga, Birang-i-Kabuli.
Rasa: Pungent, astringent.
Vīrya: Hot.
Vipāka: Pungent.
Action: Reduces fat.

Does not stimulate appetite but rather works at the tissue level and reduces fat.

Good anthelmintic. (Take 1 teaspoon of powder, this acts as a purgative, then another teaspoon. It colours the urine red).

Good against infective conditions.

Added to snuff (reduces phlegm).

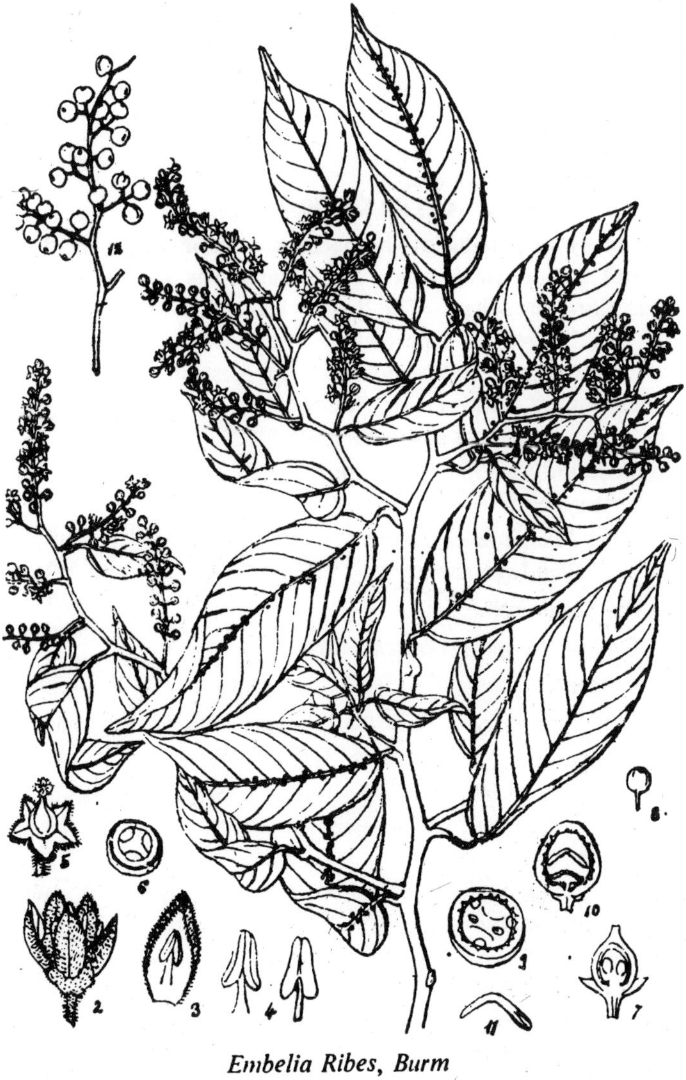

Embelia Ribes, Burm

Used as an oral contraceptive. (Old recipe: equal quantities of *Piper longum*, *Embelia ribes* and Borax. Take the 5th day after onset of period: 2 gms of powder for 7 days once daily, preferably in the morning).

There is a slightly modified modern recipe.

Use in Western medicine: As an anthelmintic, specially against tape worm.

26. CITRAKA (Plumbago)

Plumbago is a half-hardy herbaceous climbing, half-shrubby plant with a cylindrical root. The plant grows 30-110 cm high and has many branches. The lower leaves are obovate, those of the middle region lanceolate. There is a variety with red flowers and one with white flowers. An Australian variety has pale blue flowers. Flowers are followed by a capsula which is ovoide.

In medicine the red and white varieties are used, the red is the most potent.

Bot. Name: *Plumbago zeylanica*,
Plumbago rosea.

Fam.: Plumbaginaceae.

Engl.: One of the species of leadwort.

Rasa: Pungent.

Vīrya: Hot. (The plant is very hot and dry, do not
Vipāka: Pungent. use it in case of ulcers.)

Action: The red variety is used by Indian tribes as a contraceptive. The root is also used for abortion. It is irritant to the tissues.
Very appetizing, promotes intestinal digestion and tissue metabolism.
Digestive.
Emmenagogue.
Carminative.
Stops diarrhoea.
Cholagogue.
Good tonic for the liver, spleen, intestine,
Alleviates V and K.
Used against piles.

A. Plumbago Zeylanica, *Linn.* B. Plumbago Rosea, *Linn.*

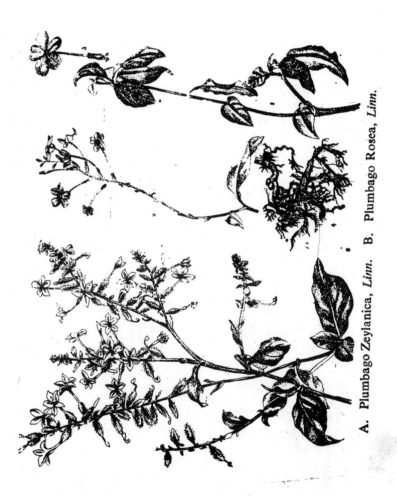

Used in Western medicine: The root of the European variety (*Plumbago europea*) is acrid and stimulates the flow of saliva when chewed. Considered to be beneficial for the relief of tooth-ache. *Plumbago zeylanica* is considered to be a strong diaphoretic.

27. KAṬUKĪ (Picorrhiza kurroa)

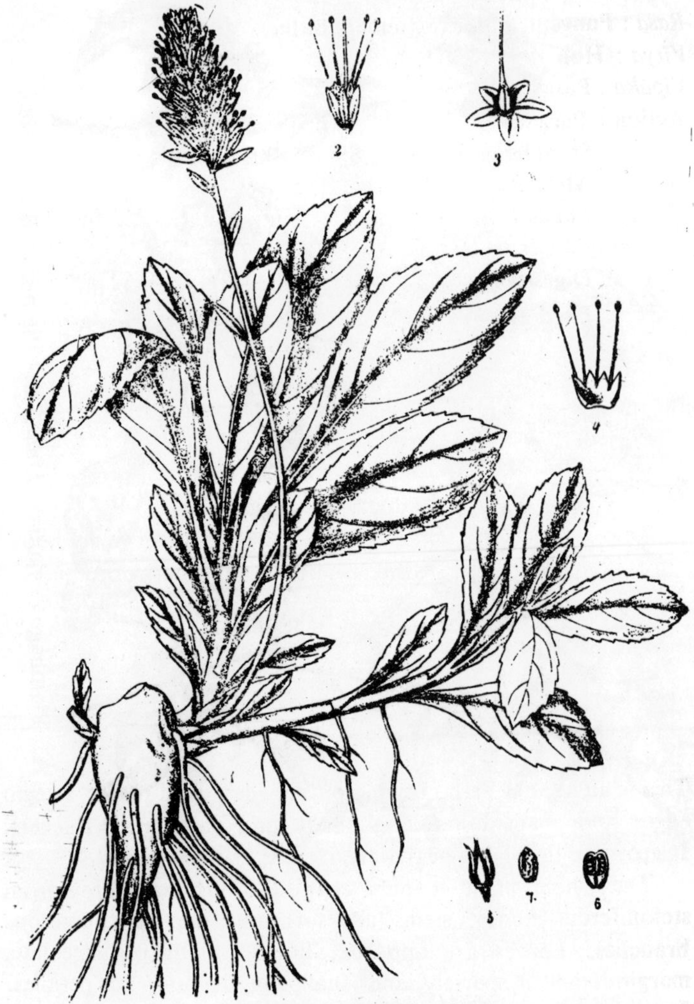

Picrorrhiza Kurroa, Benth

Picorrhiza kurroa is a plant growing at high altitudes. When the snow melts, pink flowers appear.

The plant has long rhizome and normally grows around aconite plants. Varieties of this species are abundant in Mongolia, Tibet and Bhutan.

Bot. Name: *Picorrhija kurroa.*

Fam.: Scrophulaceae.

Rasa : Pungent, bitter (extremely bitter).

Vīrya : Hot.

Vipāka : Pungent.

Action : Purgative.

Stimulates the Liver, Spleen and Gall Bladder.

Alleviates K (hot) and P (bitter).

Purifies mother's milk during lactation, if the child refuses to take it.

Digestive stimulant.

Used against : Skin diseases.

Blood impurities.

Liver defects.

Fever.

Urinary disorders.

Adiposity.

Asthma, Bronchitis.

Intestinal parasites. (Threadworm, hook-worm, round worm, tape worm etc.)

28. BHṚṄGARĀJA

This is an annual herb growing on hillsides, wild places, stream edges and roadsides among shady and damp grass thickets. It grows in the shade near water.

The whole plant is pubescent. Fibrous roots grow from stoloniferous nodes, stems are soft and fine, with numerous branches. Leaves are opposite, linear oblong or lanceolate, margin intact or sparsely and shallowly dentate, no petioles. Stem and leaves. when broken, ooze a white milky fluid which turns black. Blooms in summer, either yellowish white or blue flowers, followed by an ellipsoid flat achene. The blue flowering type is considered the best variety.

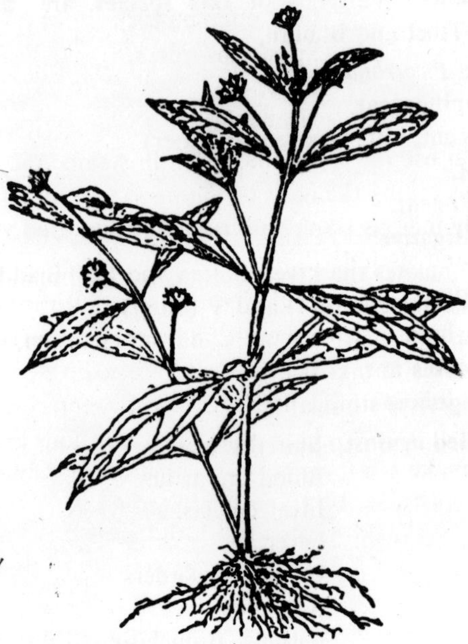

Bot. Name : *Eclipta alba.*

Fam. : Compositae.

Chinese : *Han-lien Ts'ao.*

Rasa : Pungent and bitter.

Vīrya : Hot.

Vipāka : Sweet.

Action : Well known tonic for the hair, both external and internal use.

Alleviates all three *doṣas.*

Good for skin and teeth, eyesight.

Diuretic.

Good tonic.

Used against : Cough.

Asthma.

Skin disease.

Oedema.
Anaemia.
Liver disorders (invariably added to liver compounds).
Spleen disorders.
Piles.
Headache.

For external use the species is boiled in sesame oil.

"Persons taking the juice of *Bhṛṅgarāja* only once every day and only milk as food, will live for a hundred years keeping energy and strength."

Use in Chinese medicine : Neutral, sour yet pleasant to taste. Tones the lungs, strengthens the kidneys, clears fever and detoxifies, cools the blood and stops bleeding. Used against pulmonary tuberculosis, hepatitis, gastro-enteritis, conjunctivitis, cystitis, urinary tract inflammation, boils and abscesses, poisonous snake bites, hemotysis, hematemesis, bloody stools, hematuria, epistaxis and traumatic bleeding.

29. GUḌŪCĪ

This is a perennial creeper growing wild in hedges in the shade in damp places. Subterranean root tubers, ovate rounded, frequently joined. The stem is climbing. Leaves are alternate, heart shaped, margins intact. Small white flowers in spring-summer, berry globose and red.

Bot. Name : *Tinospora cordifolia.*

Fam : Menispermaceae.

Rasa : Bitter, sweet.

Vīrya : Hot.

Vipāka : Sweet.

Action : Very good medicine for chronic fever, specially the tubercular type. Its white starch of bitter taste is good for fever. To make the starch, the stem is cut, washed and a decoction is then made. The decoction is filtered and solidified.

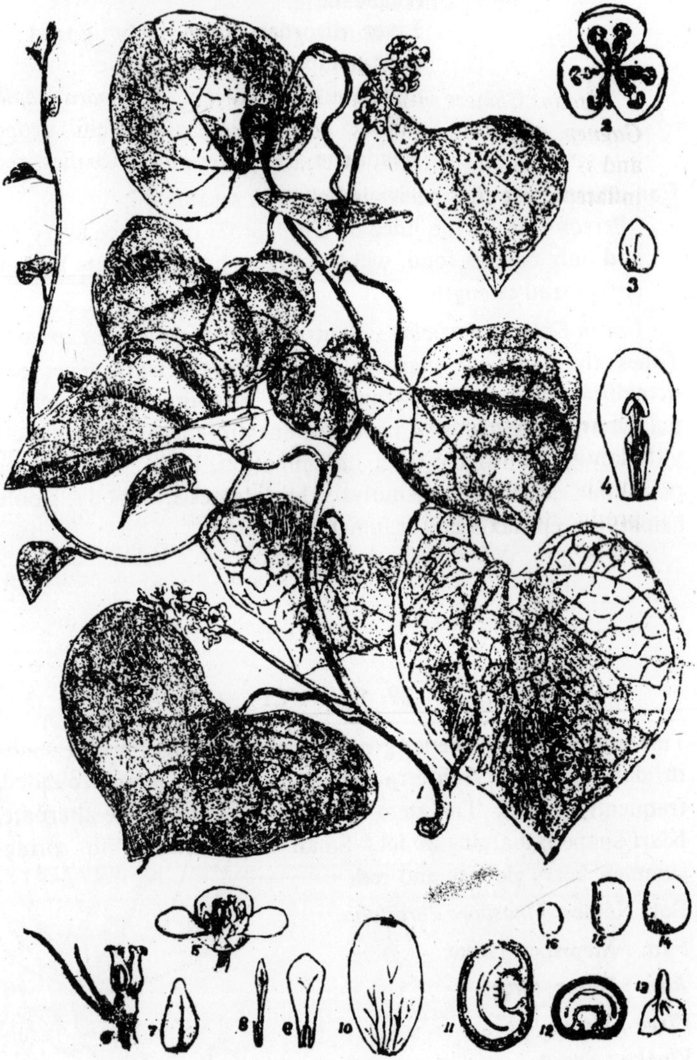

Tinospora Cordifolia, Miers

Good for liver, spleen.

Corrects mother's milk if not relished by the child.

Good diuretic.
Very mild laxative.
Used against : Malaria.
Burning sensation.
Piles.

Use in Chinese medicine : The variety *Tinospora capillipes Gagnep.* (Chin-kuo Lan) is used. This has cold-chill properties and is bitter to the taste. It clears fevers and detoxifies, reduces inflammation and alleviates pain.

30. KUMARĪ

There are several species of Aloe. They are succulent lilzaceous plants forming clusters of very fleshy leaf-blades, usually prickly at the margin and tip. The plants are either stemless or producing woody branching stems from 45 cm to 15 m tall, bearing erect spikes of yellow, orange or red flowers.

Aloes are natives of dry, sunny areas of Southern and

Two medicinal species of Aloe from Tabernaemontanus' Herbal.

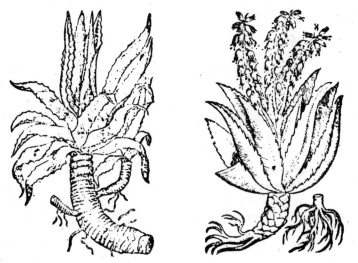

Eastern Africa. Grown in North Africa, Spain, Indonesia India and the Caribbean islands, also in Australia since recently. Aloe is not only used in India since ancient times, but also by the ancient Greeks since at least 400 B.C., as well as by the ancient Egyptians, Arabians and Chinese. The earliest recording is in the *Papyrus Ebers* of 1500 B.C.

Constituents : Barbaloin and isobarbaloin, forming "crystalline" aloin; "amorphous" aloin; aloe-emodin; resin; volatile oil.

Various species go under *Aloe vera* : *Aloe perryi baker Aloe ferox, Miller, Aloe barbadensis* etc.

Bot. Name : *Aloe barbadensis.*
Fam. : Liliaceae.
Engl. : Aloe.
German : Aloe.
Chinese : (*Aloe vulgaris*) *Lou wei* (Mandar.), *Lo woui* (Cant.)
Arabic : Sobar, Cebar.
Rasa : Bitter, Astringent, Sweet.
Vīrya : Cold.
Vipāka : Sweet.
Action : Anabolic.
Laxative.
Tonic for Liver and Spleen, specially liver stimulant.
Regulates peristaltic movements of intestines.
Good for eyesight.
Promotes digestion and relieves constipation.
Rejuvenating.
Strength giving.
Alleviates all three *doṣas*.
Carminative (good for distension of abdomen) promotes downward movement of wind in stomach.
Diuretic.
Emmenegogue.
Against : Fever,
Skin diseases,
Burns,
Ulcers,
Oedema,
Adentis,

The solidified juice of this plant is called *Musagbar*. *Kumārī-Āsava* is a useful alcoholic preparation in Āyurveda. Aloe has an effect on the Pituitary gland (anterior and posterior), the Thyroid and the Overies.

Use in Chinese medicine : Of bitter taste, non-toxic, laxative, facilitates digestion. In case of chronic constipation, amenorrhea. Chases *Yang* and *Fong* (wind). Intestinal antiparasitic. Against piles, infantile intestinal tuberculosis, convulsions, epilepsy. Chases *Yang* excess of the liver. In case of liver and eye troubles, acts upon the liver meridian, the colon meridian and heart meridian.

Use in Western medicine : As a purgative, anti-geipe medicine in connection with other carminatives, laxative, to heal burns and wounds, cuts, sunburn, as digestive, for hair and scalp care, skin care, varicose veins, psoriasis and eczematous rashes skin-cancer, ulcers, as a cleanser. Since recently again considerred a most important medicinal plant.

31. DĀḌIMA (Pomegranate)

Pomegranates have been mentioned in many ancient texts. Both the fruit-rind and the root bark were used in many ancient cultures as medicines.

The plant is a deciduous tree or shrub, about 6 m tall, with spiny tipped branches; opposite leaves, oblong or oval lanceolate, glabrous entire 2.5-6 cm long, narrowing at the base to a very short petiole.

Flowers are orange-red, waxy, 4-5 cm long and wide, they are followed by a large brownish red or yellowish edible fruit, 4-8 cm in diameter, containing numerous seeds and soft pink pulp. Widely grown in Australia.

Native to Asia, today cultivated in many countries.

Constituents : Fruit rind : yellow bitter colouring matter; gallotannic acid (30%). Root bark : alkaloids (0.9%), comprising mainly pelletierine, pseudopelletierine, isopelletierine and methylisopelletierine, to which the anthelmintic action is due; also tannins (20%). Leaf: Ursolic and betulic acids; various triterpenes.

Fruit : Invert sugar (10-20%); glucose (5-10%); citric acid (0.5-3.5%); boric acid vitamin C.

The wild variety of Pomegranate is more sour in taste, and the cultivated one more sweet.

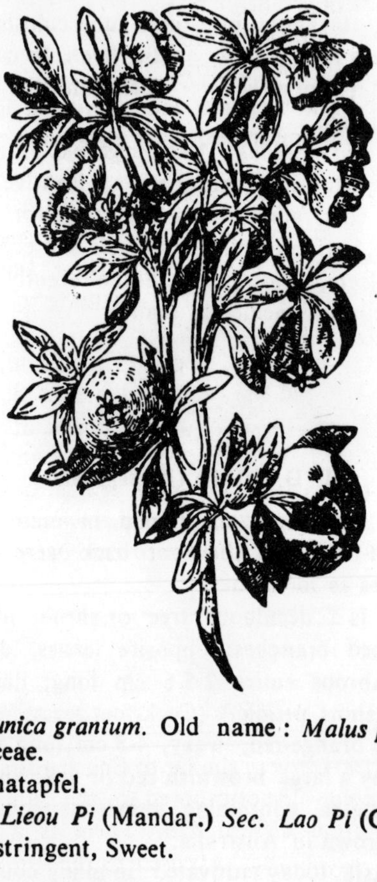

Bot. Name : *Punica grantum.* Old name : *Malus punica.*
Fam. : Punicaceae.
German : Granatapfel.
Chinese: : *Che Lieou Pi* (Mandar.) *Sec. Lao Pi* (Cant.)
Rasa : Sour, Astringent, Sweet.
Vīrya : Hot.
Vipāka : Sweet.
Action : Cardiac tonic.
Alleviates V and K if sweet, all three *doṣas*.
Aphrodisiac (the bark of the fruit).

Digestive stimulant and good action on the liver.
Carminative.
Against : Vomiting.
Diarrhoea.
Bleeding.
Internal parasites (root, which is used against tape worm).
Sprue syndrome.
Chronic colitis.

This fruit is good for pregnant ladies with a little rock salt, from the 2nd month onward, for easy pregnancy period.

Use in Chinese medicine : The bark of the fruit is used. Astringent in taste, non-toxic, intestinal antiparasitic, astringent. Against diarrhoea and dysentery, chases the *Fong* (wind) of the bones and muscles, in case of intestinal and genital haemorrhages of women, rectal prolapses. Acts upon the meridians of the colon, of the liver and the kidneys.

Use in Western medicine : The dried fruit's rind, fresh or dried root bark, fresh leaf and the fresh fruit are used. The rind is a powerful astringent used in the treatment of dysentery and diarrhoea and as an infusion for colitis and stomach ache, also as a douche in leucorrhea. The bark against tape worm (very effective when fresh) and as an emmenagogue. The leaf has antibacterial properties and is used externally for sores. The fruit is bitter and refreshing.

32. DŪRVĀ (Cocksfoot grass)

The Cocksfoot grass is very similar to Couch grass. The rhizome of this plant is used. If not exposed to the sun, this remains white, i.e. free from Chlorophyll. There is a variety which remains white, even when exposed to the sun. The plant is used in *Homa* (fire sacrifice). The juice is given to ladies for conception.

Bot. Name : *Cynodon dactylon.*
Fam. : Gramineae.
Engl. : Cocksfoot grass.

Rasa : Sweet, Bitter, Astringent.
Vīrya : Cold.
Vipāka : Sweet.
Action : Alleviates K and P.
Conception.
Against : Bleeding.
Burning sensation.
Erysipelas.

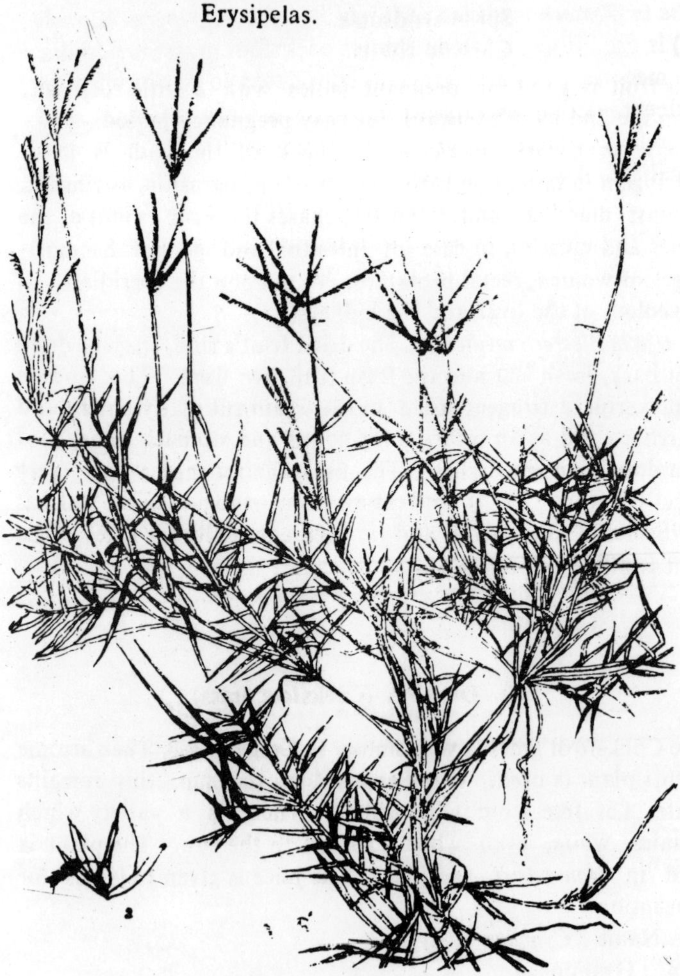

Cynodon dactylon, Pers.

Skin disease.
Ulcers.
Dysuria (as a strong diuretic).
Menorrhagea.
Piles (externally).
Insanity and Epilepsy.

Often used along with other drugs to be more effective.

Use in Western medicine : Mainly *Agropyrum repens* (Couch grass) is used instead, but in France cocksfoot grass is popular as a medicine. Couch grass is considered to be diuretic and demulcent. It palliates irritation of the urinary passages and gives relief in case of gravel. Recommended in gout and rheumatism. Used in cystitis.

33. AŚOKA

Saraca indica or *Aśoka* is a 3-4 m high bush or tree. The great Indian poet Kālidāsa describes this plant, it is also mentioned in the *Rāmāyaṇa*

Bot. Name : *Saraca indica.*

Fam. : Leguminosae.

Rasa : Astringent, Bitter.

Vīrya : Cold.

Vipāka : Sweet.

Action : Alleviates P strongly, V and K to a lesser extent.

"Useful for stopping things to go out of the body".

Bowel binding, astringent. (Astringent+cold=bowel binding).

Good for complexion.

Against : Tuberculosis.
Adenitis.
Morbid thirst.
Burning sensation.

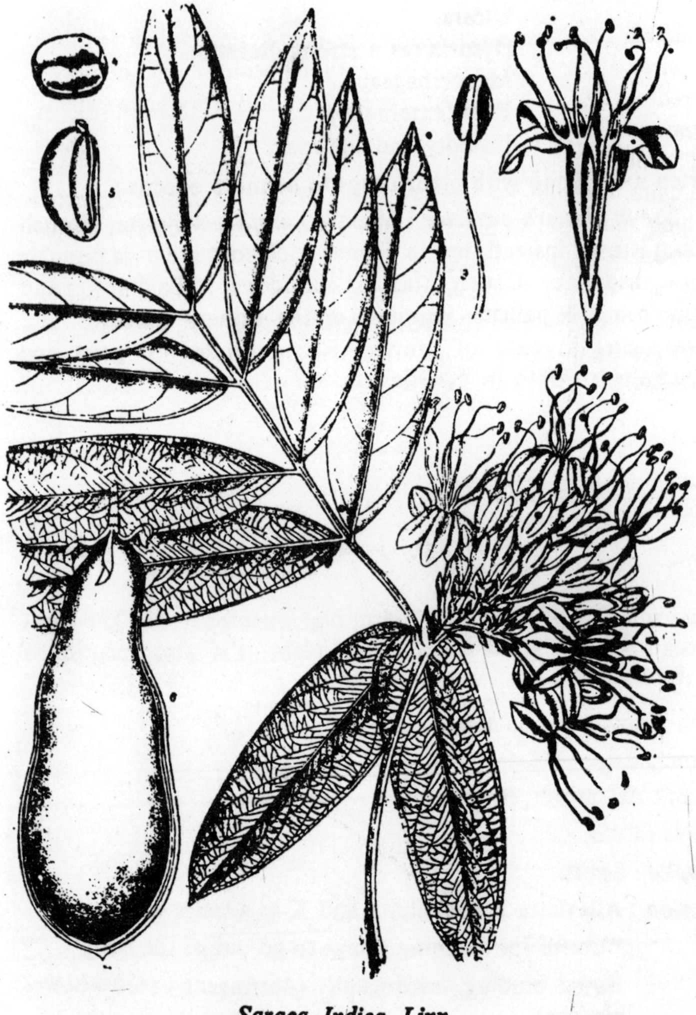

Saraca Indica, Linn

Edema.
Poisoning.
Menorrhagia.
Leucorrhea.
Pain in the uterus.

An alcoholic preparation from this plant is taken by ladies.

34. MUSTĀ

A grass-like weed with a rhizomatous root system which is thin and wiry. The root develops small, ellipsoid, naked or fibre covered tubers, these tubers have a beautiful fragrance when broken.

The plant has grass-like leaves and carries its inflorescence on a culm of triangular cross section. Three involucral bracts are long and spreading. The spikelets are from reddish-purple to brown in colour.

It is a declared noxious weed in Victoria and thought to be absent from Tasmania. The Department of Agriculture of South Australia lists it as a weed as well, to be killed by activated amitrole.

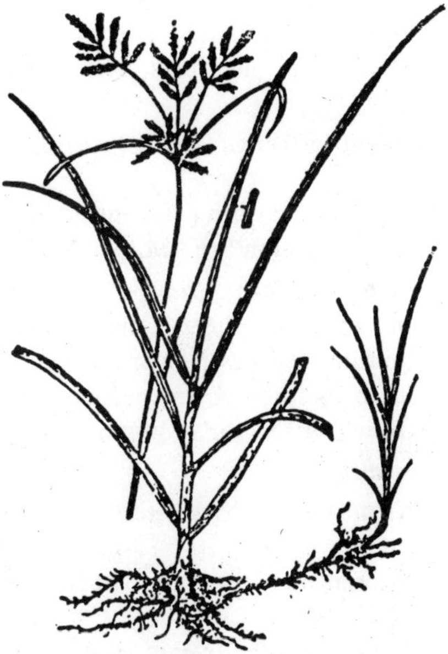

Bot Name : *Cyperus rotundus*.
Fam : Cyperaceae.
Engl. : Nut grass, Chufa, Cocograss, Motha.
Old Engl. : Galingale.
German : Runder wilder Galgan, also : wilder Galgant.

Chinese : *Hsiang-Fu.*
Rasa : Bitter, astringent, pungent.
Vīrya : Cold.
Vipāka : Pungent.
Action : Fever.
Diarrhoea.
Galactogogue (also given to animals for this purpose).
Morbid thirst.
Digestive stimulant.
Carminative.
Alleviates *Kapha, Pitta, Vāyu.*
Skin diseases.
Burning sensations, for inst. burning soles of feet.
Bleeding.
Diuretic.
Post mortem complications.

Mustā is good for children (diarahoea, colic etc.)

A syrup can be made from the tubers, boil in water, then add honey.

Mustah Arișta is an effective alcoholic drink made from this plant.

"*Mustā* is the best for causing astringent effect, promoting digestion and carmination" (FAM, p. 135).

Use in Chinese medicine : *Hsiang-Fu* is neutral, acid and slightly bitter in taste, fragrant Corrects energy circulation and relaxes congestion, restores menstrual regularity and alleviates pain, strengthens stomach and reduces distension. (Compare : "A Barefoot Doctor's Manual", p. 275).

Use in Western medicine :

According to Galen : warms dries without biting, opens, purifies, drives out.

According to Dioscurides : warms, open veins, diuretic, emmenagogue.

According to Pliny : diuretic, clears gravel. Taken in wine : strengthens stomach, is carminative, digestive, against vertigo.

According to Schroeder: Stomach, Head, Female organ. Warms and dries in the 3 degree, pungent taste, opens, carminative, against vertigo, amenorrhea and disorders caused by cold and wind.

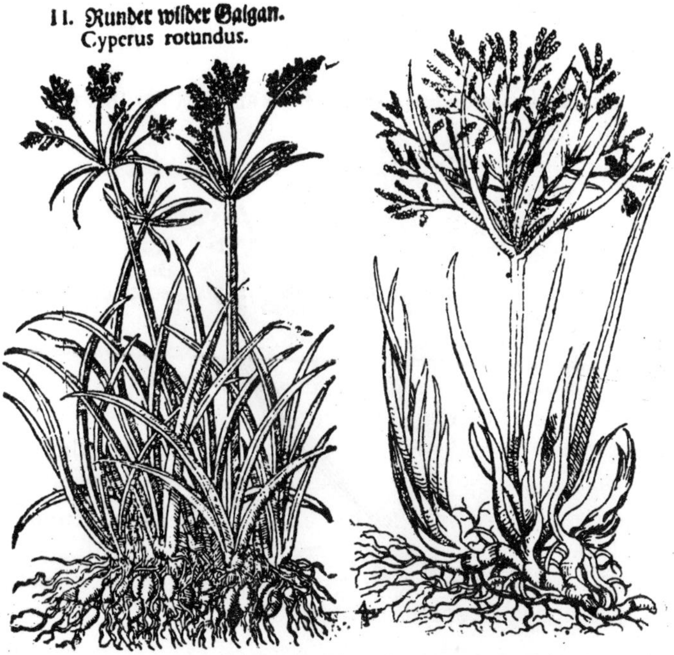
11. Runder wilder Galgan.
Cyperus rotundus.

Two classical plates of *Cyperus rotundus*. Left from 'Tabernaemontanus' "Neu voll-kommen Kräuterbuch", Offenbach 1731; right from a Francfort edition of Dioscurides of 1610.

35. GOKṢURA (Caltrops)

Caltrops is an annual herb found wild along roadsides and stream embankments. The whole plant is covered by white downy hairs. The creeping stem, multi-branching, grows as long as 1 m, it is superficially grooved. Opposite leaves, evenly pinnate compound, leaflets 5-7 pairs, long-oval shaped, margins intact. Yellow flowers in summer, followed by a globoid fruit with 2-4 spines, each containing 2-3 seeds. The spines of the fruit can puncture bicycle tyres, hence the name "puncture vine".

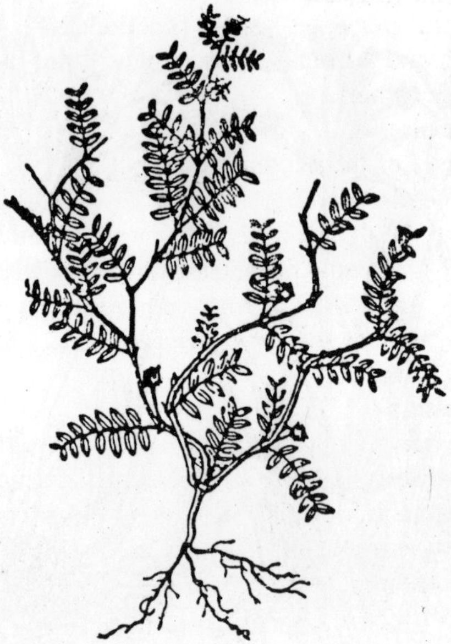

Bot. Name : *Tribulus terrestris.*
Fam. : Zygophyllaceae.
A variety which grows in sandy deserts.
Bot. Name: *Pedalium murex.*
Fam. : Pedaliaceae.
Engl. : Caltrops, Ground Burr-Nut, Puncture Vine.
Chinese : *Chi-li.*
Rasa : Sweet.
Vīrya : Cold (exeedingly cold). No action on *agnis* and enzymes, no promotion of appetite.
Vipāka : Sweet.
Action : Diuretic.
Aphrodisiac.
Nourishing.
Strength promoting.
Alleviates P and V, neutral to K.

Against : Stone in the urinary tract. (In cases of stone, first always give a strong purgative to relieve acute pain).

Diabetes (regulates kidney functions).

Cough and Asthma (water in chest), not in bronchial or allergic asthma.

Heart disease.

Diseases of the nervous system.

Uterine disorders.

Sterility. Caltrops seeds, sesame seeds and honey mixed in equal proportion and taken with goat's milk, act as a strong diuretic and anti-sterility medicine. The bigger variety is more useful in cases of sterility.

Caltrops also has rejuvenating property.

Use in Chinese medicine: Has warming properties, bitter to taste. Neutralizes the liver and dispels flatulence, clears the lungs and overcomes moisture, stimulates blood circulation.

Use in Western medicine: As an astringent, diuretic and galactogogue, (Seeds).

36. PĀṢĀṆA BHEDA

Two species of Berginea go under this name, which means "for cracking stone". The rhizome of the plant is used against stones in the urinary tract.

Bot. Name: 1st species: *Bergenea ligulata*,
2nd species: *Berginea ciliata*.

Fam.: Saxifragaceae.

Rasa: Astringent and Sweet.

Vīrya: Cold.

Vipāka: Sweet.

Pāṣāṇa Bheda is not as diuretic as *Gokṣura*, with which it is often combined, but it acts very well on stones. The rhizome of the plant is used. 1 teaspoon of the powder (*cūrṇa*) is taken twice daily, or a decoction is made of this powder.

Oxalate stones take a little more time to dissolve with this medicine, but it is very successful in cases of phosphate stones.

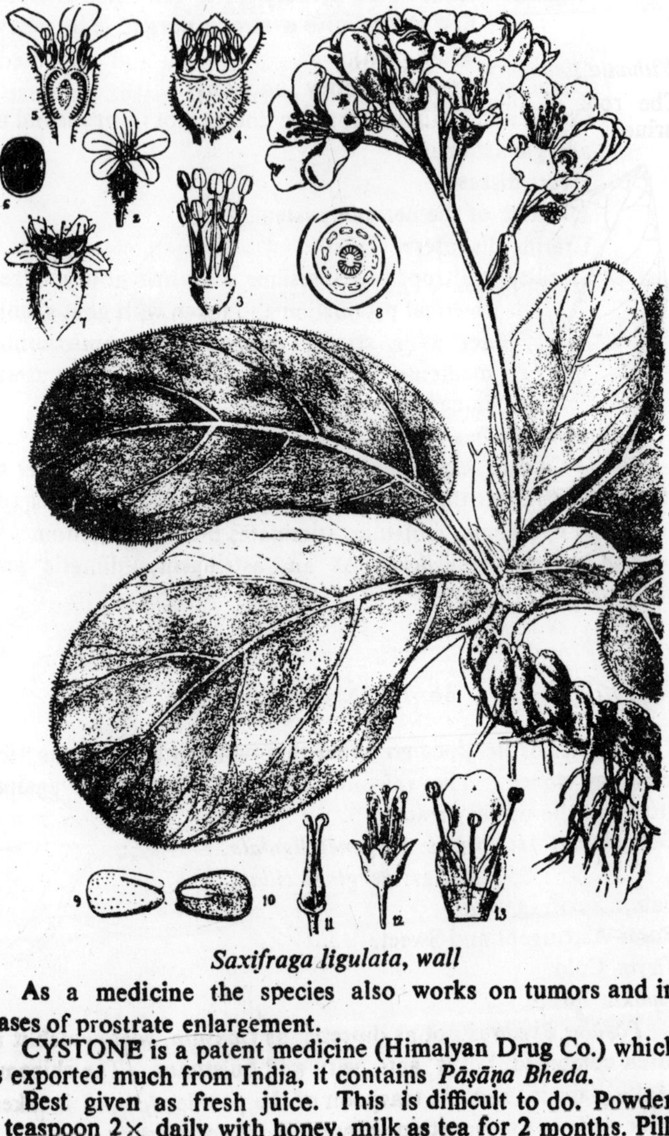

Saxifraga ligulata, wall

As a medicine the species also works on tumors and in cases of prostrate enlargement.

CYSTONE is a patent medicine (Himalyan Drug Co.) which is exported much from India, it contains *Pāṣāṇa Bheda.*

Best given as fresh juice. This is difficult to do. Powder: 1 teaspoon 2× daily with honey, milk as tea for 2 months. Pills are also available.

Bowels must be kept clear, non-wind forming diet. If diet is incorrect, the species takes much more time to work.

37. ASVAGANDHA

Withania somnifera is available as a wild plant and cultivated. The root of the wild variety smells as if soaked in horse's urine.

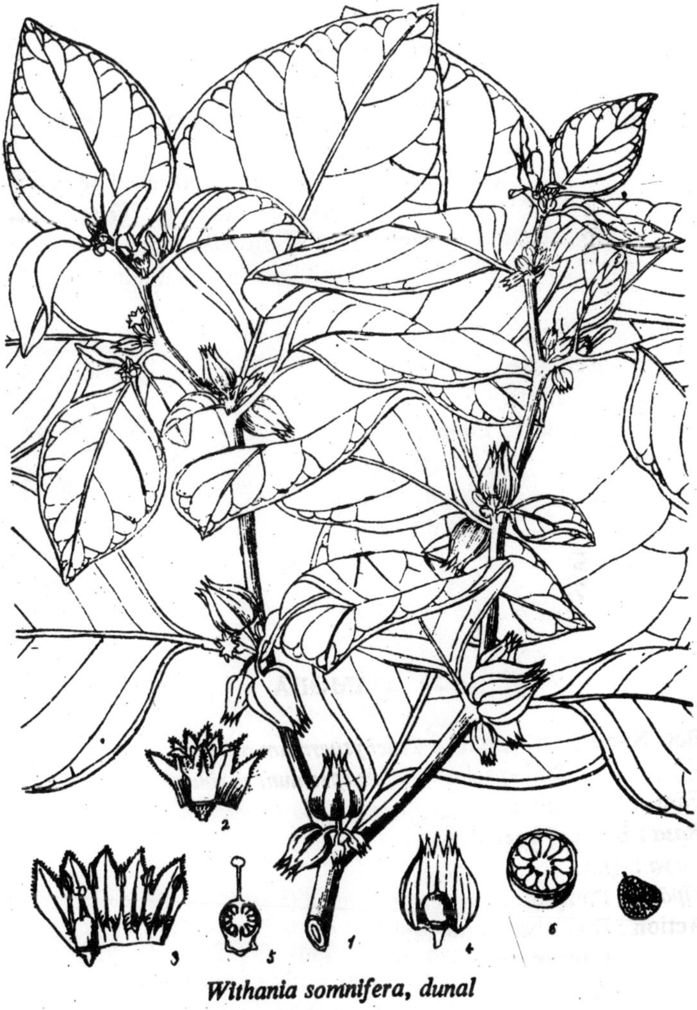

Withania somnifera, dunal

Bot. Name: ***Withania somnifera.***
Fam.: Solanaceae.

Rasa : Bitter, Astringent, Sweet.
Vīrya : Hot.
Vipāka : Sweet.
Action : Anabolic.
Nurishing and tonic.
Aphrodisiac (wild variety) (spermatopoetic=semen increasing).
(there are three categories of aphrodisiacs):
1. Stimulants.
2. Drugs increasing semen. No effect on men without sperm.
3. Drugs increasing the power of retention of semen (like nutmeg). Tests have shown that *Aśvagandha* increases sperms from 10 millions to 100 million sperms relatively.

Alleviates V and K.
Sedative.
Diuretic.
Against : Edema.
Leucoderma.
Cough.
Skin diseases.

38. AJAMODĀ

Bot. Name : 1st. species : *Trachyspermum ammi.*
2nd species : *Trachyspermum roxburghianum.*
Fam. : Umbelliferae.
Rasa : Bitter, Pungent.
Vīrya : Hot.
Vipāka : Pungent.
Action : Digestive stimulant.
Carminative.
Alleviates K, V.
Stimulates Uterus.

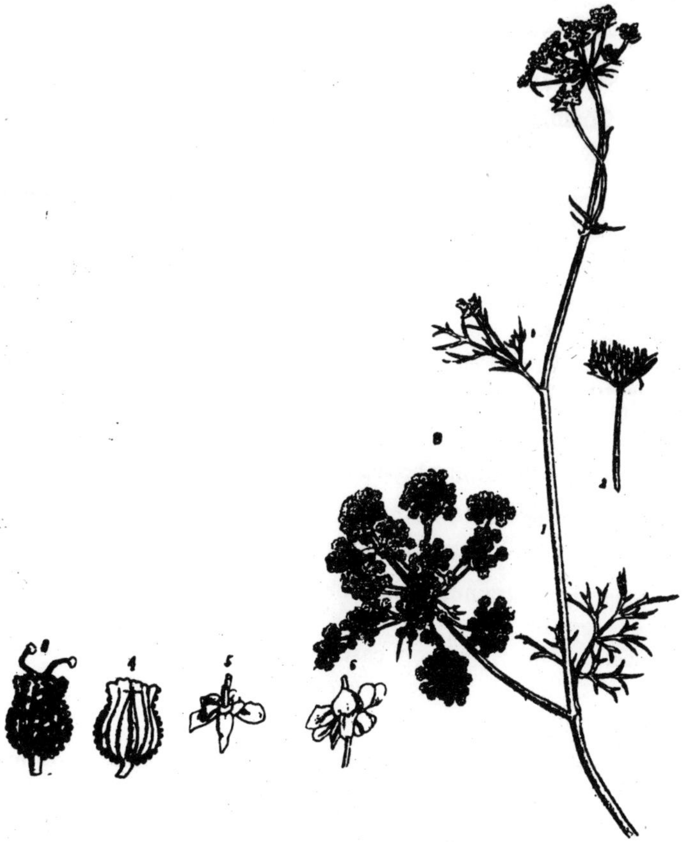

Carum Copticum, *Benth*

Reliever of colic pain. (Add rock-salt and heat in a pan).

Against : Hic-cup.
Distension of stomach.
Intestinal Parasites.
Diarrhoea.
Dysentery.
Urinary disorders.

Thymol is made from this plant. Sometimes celery seeds are taken as a substitude, but *ajamodā* is different and stronger.

39. MADHU (Honey)

Rasa : Sweet and a little astringent.

Vīrya : Cooling.

Vipāka : Sweet.

Honey reaches the finest tissues of the body and goes to the most subtle parts. It is "*yogavāha*," i.e. it enhances the therapeutic effects of drugs which are added to it.

Honey promotes intellect and strength and has many healing properties.

Alleviates all three *doṣas*, but primarily K. (Drying property).

Granulation or crystallization of honey does not alter its properties in the least, rather it is a sign of naturalness and that "not too much has been done to it".

Older honey is considered particularly valuable, specially for reducing bloodsugar in diabetes and for cough.

Sugar is contraindicated in obesity and diabetes, but pure honey can be given. In cases of obesity honey is given with hot water. This is the only case in which honey is given in hot drinks. Otherwise, honey when hot or with hot drinks is very harmful.

Indications : Ulcers (also internally against gastro-intestinal ulcers).
Bronchitis.
Asthma.
Hic-cup.
Vomiting (lemon juice with honey).
Excessive thirst (honey with lemon water).
Bleeding (also as first aid).
Diabetes.
Eye diseases, applied to eyes.

Used as a vehicle for many drugs because of its *yogavāha* character.

40. GHṚTA (Ghee)

Rasa : Sweet.
Vīrya : Cold.
Vipāka : Sweet.
Reduces all three *doṣas*, but primarily P.

Promotes longevity, good complexion, intellect, power of memory, digestive power, strength, good eyesight, but it is fattening.

Good reduction of V and P, therefore used for treatment of colic pain, (given with something hot). Promotes digestive power.

Ghee is used in cases of insanity, schizophrenia and epilepsy (the older the ghee, the better the effect. Ghee is considered old after 5 years). A few drops instilled into the nose, or a spoon taken in hot milk are effective. Old ghee is very heavy and does not promote digestion: *Triphalā Ghṛta* (*Triphalā* boiled in cow's ghee) is a special *triphalā* preparation for the eyes.

CHAPTER FOUR

Diseases and Their Treatment

1. JVARA (Fever)

In Western Medicine Fever is defined in two ways :

1. Elevation of the body temperature above the normal; in human beings above the average value of 37°C orally.
2. A disease whose distinctive feature is elevation of body temperature.

In Āyurvedic Medicine the second category would be a more adequate description of *Jvara*, in fact, a group of diseases falls under this category. The state of fever is not only limited to mammals, but also to other animals, plants and even to a pond. *Jvara* can be caused by 8 factors, i.e. it can be of 8 different types :

1. V.
2. P.
3. K.
4. VP.
5. VK.
6. PK.
7. S. (*sānnipātika*, i.e. VPK)
8. Caused by external factors (injuries, germs, affliction by "supernatural" bodies, grief, anger, passion.

Jvara is thus caused by aggravation of 1, 2 or 3 *doṣas* or by external factors.

Origin

First the *agnis* in the stomach become affected, the stomach is the *udbhavasthāna* (site of origin). The affected *agnis* are then carried by a *Rasa Dhātu* channel to the site of manifestation: the skin.

Generally there is a little or no sweating during fever. If the patient is made to sweat, the fever is reduced.

Symptoms

The patient suffers from general malaise, there is loss of appetite and a tendency of lacrimation. According to the type of fever the signs and symptoms differ.

V type : much pain all over the body.

P type : high temperature, burning sensation.

K type : lower temperature but congestion, cough, cold, constipation, loss of appetite.

Treatment

1. Give rest to the stomach. Fasting is an excellent treatment, allow the patient to fast or miss meals. If the patient is hungry, as in P type of fever, give light food. Give much boiled water (this is light for digestion), add ginger, long pepper or pepper to this water.

   Frequent urination will eliminate *āma*.
2. Stimulate digestion by giving digestive stimulants (ginger, long pepper, black pepper). Dry ginger powder with honey, turmeric powder with warm milk.

   At the end of the fever, give a light purgative.

   No yoghurt should be permitted during fever.

If the *Jvara* is of the K type, no sleep during the day is permitted, since this aggravates K and *āma*.

If V is aggravated : ginger powder with ghee.

If P is aggravated : ginger powder with butter.

If K is aggravated : give honey by itself or mixed with ginger powder, or also with *Tulasi* or Mint varieties.

Special Medicines

Mṛtyuñjaya Rasa. Consists principally of Mercury, Sulphur, Aconite and Borax, Aconite combined with Borax has no adverse effect on the body.

2. KĀSA (Cough, Bronchitis)

A condition, transient or chronic, in which persistent irritation of respiratory mucosa give rise to episodes of coughing.

Kāsa is of 5 types :

1. V.
2. P.
3. K.
4. *Kṣataja* (produced by injuries).
5. *Kṣayaja* (produced by loss, reduction).

The types 4 and 5 are produced by aggravation of all the 3 *doṣas*.

Kāsa can be caused by exposure to smoke, dust, excess of exercise, ununctuous food, repression of natural urges.

Origin

Originates in the stomach. Channels carry *rasa* to the site of manifestation : lungs or throat. K is involved in the pathogenesis. Pressure from below causes the sound of a broken bronze vessel (*kāṁsya*=bronze). From this the term *kāsa* is derived.

Symptoms

V : Cardiac pain, pain in chest, face has a tired look, loss of strength, patient cannot speak, frequent urge for coughing, cough is dry.

P : Burning sensation in chest, dry mouth, desire to drink water, sometimes vomiting of yellow material, patient looks pale, burning sensation in the body.

K : Sticky mouth, headache, body is feeling heavy like full of phlegm, itching, anorexia, not many attacks of cough, but when coughing, a lot of phlegm comes out.

Kṣataja : Can be caused by excessive sex, carrying heavy weight etc. because breath is held during these activities. Continuous coughing, blood spitting, pain in finger joints, hoarse voice, thirsty, "voice like a pigeon".

Kṣayaja : (*kṣaya*=reduction), caused by unwholesome food and insufficient exercise, suppression of natural urges, hateful disposition, snobbishness. Pain all over the body, burning sensation, dry cough, weakness, reduction of muscle tissue, spits blood and pus. This is the borderline to tuberculosis.

Treatment

Because of its origin in the stomach : fasting or taking of barley gruel, fasting should not be carried out in the 4th and 5th types *Kāsa* (VP and VK). In this case meat soups may be given, these are light for digestion and nourishing.

In the case of diseases originating in the stomach, emetic therapy is effective.

In cases of *kāsa,* 2 days after origin, emetic therapy is carried out. This is particularly effective in K types of *kāsa.* Emetic therapy is not carried out in case of *kṣataja* type of *kāsa* (because of lung injuries), neither is it desirable in *kṣayaja kāsa* cases.

Don't give yoghurt, sour fruits or fruit juice, instead give sweet fruit juice, milk and oat gruel, cheese, bread and milk.

Water is given boiled, cold or luckewarm. Water can also be boiled with ginger, black pepper or long pepper.

V type : medicated ghee with long pepper, ginger.

P type : medicated butter.

Special Medicines

Dry grapes (raisins) are very good, also the alcoholic drink prepared from them. This is called *Drākṣa Āsava.* To this are added pepper, black pepper etc.

In K conditions : *Lakṣmī Vilāsa* and *Nāradīya Lakṣmī Vilāsa,* or also *Mahā Lakṣmī Vilāsa,* which also contains gold in *bhasma* form. In case of V.P. types : ordinary *Lakṣmī Vilāsa. Acacia catechu* together with a little camphor, very effective as lozenges. For sweeter taste a little liquorice may be added.

• *Sitopalādi Cūrṇa,* which is made in the following way :

Take sugar powder 16 parts,

Bamboo salt 8 parts. (this substance which is found inside mature bamboo, is not a salt but a rather tasteless substance, good for Ca deficiency),

Long pepper 4 parts,

Cinnamon 2 parts,

Cardamom seed 1 part,

First powder the ingredients separately, then mix :

In V. P. type : with honey and ghee.

In K type : with honey alone.

In types 4 and 5 (VP, VK) : with honey and ghee. (Don't take this powder dry).

Take for 6-7 days.

Turmeric powder is also very good for *kāsa*.

3. ŚVĀSA ROGA (Asthma)

Śvāsa actually means "breathing in and out"; *śvāsa roga* is asthma.

According to Āyurveda there are 5 varieties of asthma : *Mahā śvāsa*, *Ūrdhva śvāsa*, *Chinna Śvāsa*, *Tamaka śvāsa* and *Kṣudra śvāsa*.

The first sign of all of these is invariable : breathing problems.

Origin

Asthma originates in the stomach. Passes through channels carrying *rasa*, gets located in lungs.

Now the 5 types in detail.

1. *Mahā Śvāsa*. (Great or serious asthma). Signs and symptoms : the patient, when breathing, feels pain and discomfort, is not satisfied with deep breathing, there is loss of consciousness, eyes move from side to side, cannot close mouth, obstructed passages of urine and stool, unable to speak. This is a dangerous situation.
2. *Ūrdhva Śvāsa*. (Upwards asthma). Signs and symptoms: The patient can exhale, but cannot inhale properly, so there is lack of oxygen for the brain and heart. The patient looks upward, eyes roll here and there, there is great pain in the chest and the head, patient does not

want to live or do anything. If neglected, he may die.

3. *Chinna Śvāsa.* (Broken asthma), Signs and symptoms: Broken respiration which suddenly stops. Excrutiating pain in the chest, tympanitis (distension of abdomen from accumulation of gas), perspiration, eyes fixed, patient becomes emaciated, vascularization takes place (bleeding from eyes etc.).

4. *Tamaka Śvāsa.* (Allergic asthma). When V, instead of going down, goes up, it makes the head and the neck stiff, K is aggravated., this results in rhinitis, beginning like an attack of cold. Thereafter obstruction of respiration results and a kind of "*gharghar*" sound results. The patient gets excrutiating pain in the head and chest, often he becomes unconscious. There is dry cough, when phlegm is thrown out, the patient feels relief. The throat is sore, the patient is incapable of sleeping, will not sleep on his back but in a bent position. There is desire for hot things (fomentations, drinks). The conditions get aggravated with cold wind from the seaside. If the patient is strong, it is curable in the early stage, afterwards it becomes difficult. In the early morning the patient will spit, when conditions have become chronic. Sometimes *Tamaka śvāsa* has a P involvement. If P is involved with V and K there is burning sensation, the patient faints, food is not digested. This type of asthma is alleviated by cold things like water and cold wind.

5. *Kṣudra Śvāsa* (Minor type of asthma). Because of much unctuous food and suppression of natural urges, this minor type of asthma may result. It is easily cured.

Treatment

In treatment the stomach has to be corrected and breathlessness be taken care of, i.e. the site of origin and the site of manifestation have to be taken care of.

Hic-cup, Bronchitis and Asthma have almost identical treatment. If bronchitis or allergic rhinitis are not treated, the conditions may lead to asthma.

There may be hereditary tendencies to asthma. Traditionally it is believed that indiscriminate killing of animals leads to asthma in future births.

Premonitory signs are always pain in the cardiac region, constipation, all connected with the stomach and V. *Prāṇa vāyu* and *udāna vāyu* get obstructed by K.

Always take care of K and V during treatment. To alleviate K and V the "three pungent drugs" are useful. In chronic stages we give long pepper. Simultaneously to promote strength. Honey is useful for this, since it also acts against K. *Hiṅgu* (Asafoetida) brings V downwards.

Treatment always begins by correcting the stomach and K excess. If the stomach is stimulated (vagus nerve, parasympathetic) there is a sympathetic reflex in the lungs, mucus comes out. Obstructions in channels of circulation have to be cleared.

Vomiting is useful to break the pathogenesis. Next important step; *bowels should be clear*. Remove constipation by a purgative or laxative, even if patients do not feel constipated. Conditions are aggravated by psychic factors. Give light food and avoid indigestion, regulate motions to be a little more frequent than normal.

Special Medicines

A powder to be taken at night consists of 3 parts *Harītakī*+1 part rock-salt. (adding rock-salt to *Harītakī's* 5 tastes means to add the 6th (saline) taste to the preparation). This powder clears the bowels. *Harītakī* is hot and has special action on the lungs and the heart. This way the disease is corrected.

If there is more of phlegm : mix *Harītakī* and old jaggery (1 yearld old or more) in equal quantity, take at bed-time and in the morning.

If K is more aggravated : prescribe ginger powder and jaggery in equal quantity. Jaggery by itself is good for asthma.

In cases of bronchial asthma caused by allergy : turmeric is given in different forms. Fry 4-5 teaspoons of turmeric with 1 teaspoon of butter, add a little jaggery or sugar powder, give 3-5 times for acute attack.

Cyavanaprāśa is good for asthma.

ŚVĀSA KUṬHĀRA (lit. : Asthma-Axe) :

Mercury 1 pt.

Sulphur 1 pt.

Aconite 1 pt.

Borax 1 pt.

Realgar (arsenic) 1 pt (red arsenic).

Black pepper 8 pts.

Three pungent drugs 8 pts.

Mercury and Sulphur are triturated first, they become black and there is no more glaze. Trituration continues for 7 days. Then the Aconite root and Borax are added in the following way : the Borax is calcined over fire, take this powder and add to the Aconite pieces, which have previously been soaked in virgin cow's urine or milk. This will be sticky. Now the arsenic is added, then black pepper is added, one globule after the other, triturate. It takes about 3 months to get all fully powdered. Finally add the other drugs.

Use in dose of 125 mg, adults upto 250 mg, twice in 24 hours.

Ginger juice+honey will melt phlegm.

VĀSĀRIṢṬA. (+*Dhūtura*). Two teaspoons of this relieves, but it has a very drying effect on the body. Therefore do not give this *Āsava* with *Dhatūra* if there is dry cough, but only *Vāsāriṣṭa*.

Vāsa (leaves)+*Dhatūra* (leaves or seeds) made into an asthma cigarette, or burnt in a vessel and thus inhaled, gives temporary relief.

CANDRĀMṚTA (Moon-Nectar) will make phlegm come out.

To this *bhasma* of mica (*Abhraka bhasma*) can be added. This is prepared by putting mica to the fire 100 times. Add 125 mg.

If there is still no relief, add a little peacock feather *bhasma.*

If the patient is completely emaciated: give *Śvās a Cintāmaṇi,* which contains gold along with the substances described.

Remember that

Physician Drugs Attendants Patient	all 4 are involved in healing.
Strong will power Wealth Obedience	on the part of the patient are necessary for recovery.

Diet for Asthma

Any diet which is sweet or which is sour will aggravate K, therefore it is of no use. K is present in the pathogenesis.

Pungent, bitter and astringent properties should be given to the patient.

The channels of circulation must not be obstructed, therefore avoid yoghurt, sour fruits and their juices and also bananas.

Sweet things which do not aggravate K can be given in small quantities : sugar, rice, chick-peas.

Wheat is best for asthma patients.

Cow's milk is good, but goat milk is better in this case. Give plenty of goat's milk. Don't use cold things, and always give freshly prepared food.

Buttermilk can be given since it is the reverse of yoghurt in action.

4. AJĪRṆA (Indigestion). AGNIMĀNDYA (Suppression of the Power of Digestion).

Causes

Wrong diet, drinks and regimens.

Sleep during the day is not permitted in such cases, sleep after taking meals leads to *āma* formation.

Various psychic factors before, during and after taking food are involved. The *agnis* are affected. (1 in intestines, 5 in liver and 7 in tissues). If possible keep the mind calm after taking food, avoid agitation.

V, P, K type. Normally, in case of suppression of *agnis*, there is much K. But there are all three types.

V : wind in stomach and pain.

P : acid eructation, restlessness of mind and pungent taste in the mouth.

K : Laziness, no desire for work and *āma* formation.

Treatment

Take ginger and rock-salt before taking food.

Sour, saline and pungent things are recommended. All of these contain *agni-mahābhūta*. Powder of the seeds of sour pomegranate is Good. The powder is dried up and a little salt and cummin seed is added.

Hiṅgvaṣṭaka Cūrṇa, a preparation of Asafoetida and 7 other drugs, is useful.

P type : give a little ghee, which will relieve the burning sensation and relieve P condition.

K type : give ginger, also before food.

V type : Asafoetida brings down V.

Piper nigrum and *Piper longum* also help.

Yoghurt is taken with cummin seeds and salt, add ginger. (Give yoghurt only if there is no asthma or cold at the time, neither in cases of rheumatism).

For constipated patients yoghurt+salt+cummin seeds are excellent during day meals, but not at night. *Harītakī* chewed with a little lemon, before or after meals is also useful.

5. ĀMAVĀTA (Rheumatism)

The 1st stage in children involves fever and a little pain in the joints. Gradually the heart is affected.

The 2nd stage affects several joints in adults Osteoarthritis, rheumatoid arthritis and gout as well as spondylosis are included.

Causative factors

Unwholesome foods and regimens, bad digestive power, insufficient exercise, too much unctuous food and too much meat—all this leads to *āma* formation.

Site of Origin

Mainly the colon, but the whole intestinal tract is involved, right from the formation of saliva to the rectum.

Through eating of contradictory food and mental tension V is aggravated in the colon. Psychic factors help in the formation of *āma*, which is then carried out of the place of origin.

Āma and V together affect the *agnis*, and finally there is *āma* formation at every level.

The *āma* gets lodged in the joints and the heart. The *Rasavāha Srotas* act as transport channel.

Signs and Symptoms

Malaise, anorexia, lethargy, fever, indigestion, swellings in different parts of the body. Joints are affected, bones, cervical vertebra, thorasic vertebra, hip bones, scapula bones and others are affected.

V is aggravated (this is ununctuous). Normally for curing V aggravation we give oil, also ghee. But these are heavy for digestion and therefore tend to aggravate *āma* in case of rheumatic disorders. To reduce *āma*, we therefore give ununctuous things. Select such drugs to reduce *āma* and V. If rheumatism is caused by aggravation of:

V : there is excruciating pain in the joints, rough skin, stomach distension and indigestion.

P : there is burning sensation all over the body, specifically in joints.

K : the patient slowly becomes crippled.

In the early morning there often is a little pain in the heel, because the *āma* gets moving in the morning.

In osteoarthritis, where *āma* formation is negligible, there is pain when moving.

Treatment

Fasting. Do not advise fasting in excess, since this would aggravate V too much.

Medicines which are bitter in taste (These alleviate V and *āma*, although V may be slightly aggravated).

Pungent things. (this may again aggravate V, but first the *āma* has to be attacked and reduced).

Since *āmavāta* is a disease (or group of diseases) of the large intestine : give purgatives, or also medicated enema.

Medicines should be pungent, hot, digestion stimulating. Therefore give :

Ginger which is pungent and reduces *āma*.

Turmric. Give this fried in ghee because its nature by itself is ununctuous.

Ajamodā.

Garlic. This is pungent and has 5 tastes, and it is hot in potency.

Ginger Paste may be applied hot.

Harītakī is suitable because it is hot.

Semecarpus anacardium, oriental cashew nut, is a useful drug. It is also used for leucoderma and cancer. The drug is a little poisonous and some are allergic to it (it may cause itching). A jam or a powder prepared from it is therefore taken along with ghee, so that it will not touch the mucous membrane of the mouth. If a reaction occurs this will be over in one day.

Guggulu (*Commiphora mukul*) is very useful. The gum from this tree is collected by injuring the stem. The gum is also used for incense. The actual medicine is prepared as follows: first a decoction of *triphalā* is prepared, then the gum is added to it, it will melt. All is then strained and the liquid put into another vessel. This liquid is then boiled further till it becomes semi-solid. Finally it is put into the sun and dried. It looks like the gum of almond trees.

The gum thus prepared is used for cholesterol excess, disorders of the genitory tract, urinary trouble and rheumatism.

By adding a purgative it can be made even more effective

for instance it can be triturated with raw castor oil (the refined type is less active). This will be very purgative. To this purified Sulphur, a little ginger powder isa dded.

Here follows a recipe of a medicine known as *Siṃhanāda Guggulu:*

Triphalā 150 gms
Sulphur (purified) 50 gms
Guggulu (purified gum) 50 gms
Castor oil 50 gms
Ginger powder 50 gms

Prepare according to the method indicated above in an iron vessel. (This is specified). Some of these preparations also contain a little iron in *bhasma* form (against anaemia). There is also *Yogarāja* or *Mahāyogarāja Guggulu* without castor oil for weak and sensitive patients.

Castor oil seeds, when green on the tree, can be given along with milk as a purgative.

Diet and Regimens

The patient should not sleep in the day, specially after taking food.

Avoid food which is heavy for digestion. Don't give much unctuous food.

No pulses, no rice. Give barley, oats, wheat instead. Vegetable (leafy) of bitter taste are good. Garlic and turmeric are given. Avoid yoghurt and Seafish. Don't expose the patient to cold wind. Avoid stress. Avoid mutually contradictory foods and drinks (boiled honey). Don't suppress natural urges (motions).

Apply medicated oils externally (some of these contain *Dhatūra* or Belladonna, usually the oils are vasodilating).

Pañca Karma Therapy

Before the actual *Pañca Karma* treatment *Snehana* (oleation and *Svedana* (sweating) are prescribed. For the oleation medicated ghee is drunk, this will dislodge *āma* and make it soft. Then give the fomentations (*Svedana*) of which there are 13 types.

Once dislodged, the *āma* comes to the intestines. Allow it to flow back to the intestinal tract. Then the 5 therapies are applied. The patient will become weak and there is a special food regimen to be observed during the treatment for 7 days.

There is a violent shake up of the nervous system during the treatment and no work can be carried out by the patient. Now the actual 5 therapies (*Pañca Karma*):

1. *Vamana* (Emetic). This is radical, upto the point when bile comes out. Not in case of heart problem.
2. *Virecana* (Purgative), till mucus material comes out.
3. *Nirūha Basti* (decoctions, if *āma vāyu*).
4. *Anuvāsana Basti* (oil, if *nirāma vāyu* condition).
5. *Nasya* (Inhalation therapy).

For permanent conditions different recipes are used.

6. PRAMEHA

(*A Group of Obstinate Urinary Diseases, including Diabetes*)

Prameha, sometimes simply called *Meha*, is a group of twenty obstinate urinary diseases.

In 10 out of these 20, K is prominently involved in the pathogenesis.

In 6 out of these 20, P is prominently involved in the pathogenesis.

In 4 out of these 20, V is prominently involved in the pathogenesis.

Causative Factors

Too much sedentary habit and no physical work.

Inability to sleep or too much sleep.

Excessive consumption of yoghurt.

Much eating of the flesh of animals living in water and marsh.

Eating freshly harvested rice or wheat. (Freshly harvested rice is rich in *Jala-Mahābhūta*).

Excessive consume of starch, specially in refined food, leads to diabetes. (For this reason diabetes is also called "rich man's disease" in India).

Mental worries and stress in excess can lead to diabetes as well.

During the pathogenesis *Medas* as well as the muscle

tissues and "sticky material" (including sweat) get affected inside the body, this produces diabetes.

The 10 types of K *Prameha* are relatively easy to cure. (Give pepper and turmeric, which reduce K, fat and muscle).

The 6 types of P *Prameha* are more difficult to cure. Drugs which are hot in *vīrya* and pungent in *vipāka* should be given. In this case there is a feeling of dirt in the mouth and bad smell, desire to clean the teeth and the mouth, which is sticky. There is burning sensation in the body or only in the skin, much thirst and sweet taste in the mouth).

The 4 types of V *Prameha* are difficult and often very difficult to cure. Since V is ununctuous, give oils and sweet things, these aggravate K however. There are relatively few medicines which alleviate V + K, but turmeric and *āmalakī* will alleviate both V and K.

The 10 Types of K Prameha

1. *Udaka-Meha* (Water-*Meha*). This is actually a very minor type of diabetes insipidus. During this more urine is passed like water.
2. *Ikṣu-Meha* (Sugarcane-*Meha*), sugarcane diabetes, which is mainly caused by the liver.
3. *Sāndra-Meha* (Density-*Meha*), there is thicker urine discharge, but no sugar is present in it.
4. *Surā-Meha* (Alcohol-*Meha*), the urine has the smell and appearance of alcohol.
5. *Piṣṭa-Meha* (Paste or Dough-*Meha*), the urine will have much solid material as if it would contain some dough or paste. Albumen and phosphate are present in the urine.
6. *Śukra-Meha* (Semen-*Meha*), the urine will appear as if it had semen in it, sometimes semen is present. In this case, often there is a prostrate problem, Leucorrhea in the case of women.
7. *Sikatā Meha* (Sand or Small gravel-*Meha*), there seems to be sand or gravel in the urine, solid discharges of various kinds.
8. *Śīta-Meha* (Cold-*Meha*), the urine is excessively cold.
9. *Śanair-Meha* (Small-*Meha*), the patient passes small quantities of urine frequently.

10. *Lālā-Meha* (Saliva-*Meha*), the urine is like mucus or saliva.

The 6 Types of P Prameha

1. *Kṣāra-Meha* (Caustic or Salty-*Meha*) the urine has an alkaline consistency and taste.
2. *Haridrā-Meha* (Turmeric-*Meha*), the urine is very yellow like turmeric. The urine is also very yellow in case of jaundice. But in the case of *Haridrā-Meha* the liver is not affected.
3. *Mañjiṣṭhā-Meha* (*Mañjiṣṭhā* is a red plant), occasionally there is blood in the urine.
4. *Rakta-Meha*, this is Haematuria, blood is present in the urine.
5. *Nīla-Meha* (Blue-*Meha*), the urine is bluish or indigo in colour.
6. *Kāla-Meha* (Black-*Meha*), the urine is blackish.
   All these 6 types require much effort to cure.

The 4 Types of V Prameha

1. *Vasā-Meha* (Liquid Fat-*Meha*), a lot of fat will pass with the urine. Serious.
2. *Majjā-Meha* (Marrow-*Meha*), much uric acid, urates etc. passed in excess.
3. *Madhu-Meha* (Honey-*Meha*), this is diabetes mellitus. The cells in the islets of Langerhans in the pancreas are damaged in this case. The normal insulin mechanism is disturbed. For this disease see explanations further down.
   All three *doṣas* together can cause *Madhu-Meha*.
4. *Hasti-Meha* (Elephant-*Meha*), there is a "waterfall" of urine, large quantities of urine are passed, but there is no sugar presence. This is diabetes insipidus of serious nature. It is palliable, but difficult to cure.

Diabetes can be hereditary as well as acquired. Fat people get it more easily than thin people. Severe hereditary cases are often practically incurable.

10 types of carbuncles are caused by diabetes.

Diabetes is a disease characterized by the habitual discharge of large quantities of urine and by excessive thirst. It is of

2 kinds: diabetes insipidus and diabetes mellitus. In the case of diabetes insipidus there is excessive urination but the urine is free from sugar. In case of diabetes mellitus there is chronic disorder of the carbohydrate metabolism due to disturbance of normal insulin mechanism.

Due to the impairment of sugar metabolism the tissue cells do not get enough material for the production of energy. This results in weakness of the patients. Overnourished people easily get affected by this disease. Higher blood sugar levels lead to many complications like coma, carbuncles etc.

The pancreas, the kidneys and the liver are affected in diabetes.

Line of Treatment for Diabetes

The body fat of the patient has to be reduced and the function of the pancreas has to be regulated to promote sugar metabolism.

Bitter things have to be given as food, specially *Karela* (bitter gourd). The juice of the leaves and the fruits of the plant is used in a dose of one ounce, twice daily, preferably on empty stomach. Bitter things will work on fat, K and muscle tissue. (Bitter taste is formed by *Vāyu* and *Ākāśa Mahābhūta*).

The patient's habits have to be changed and stress is to be avoided, reduce mental worries.

Chicory and coffee can be given, although coffee brings stress, but coffee is better than tea and alcohol in this case.

Recommended are chick-peas, ununctuous food and less of sugar, but do not take saccharine.

1. Regulate the kidneys, the pancreas and the liver, tone up these.

2. Give turmeric, *āmalakī*, *guggulu* and *śilājatu*. (of *śilājatu* half a teaspoon in milk on empty stomach).

śilājatu is exuded from stones in high altitude when these are exposed to the sun..

It is a kind of gum of stones, in English it is also known as asphalt. The *śilājatu* from the Himalayas is famous, it is eaten by rats and monkeys also.

To obtain it, the stones are broken and boiled in water. In this way a kind of cream forms. This layer of cream is taken out and dried in the sun. The stones used are black greasy. *Śilājatu* smells like cow's urine.

If the stones contain gold, gold-*śilājatu* is obtained, if they contain copper, copper-*śilājatu* is obtained. *Śilājatu* works well on diabetes.

Śilājatu is also a strong aphrodisiac.

Śilājatu together with *guggulu* is given in cases of fractures. It goes to the joints and forms a callus quickly.

Śilājatu and *guggulu* together are also used in case of osteoarthritis, spondylosis.

Candraprabhā is a pill containing camphor, *śilājatu* and *guggulu*.

Avoid sugar and much starch like rice, potato, banana, cereals containing much carbohydrate, also fat, oil. Neem leaves are good. These, when taken in the morning, reduce blood sugar. Certain yogic *asanas* also reduce diabetes in the early stages.

Saptaraṅga is a wood with separate layers, with which scientific experiments are carried out in India. This is also very effective in reducing the blood sugar level.

Useful are also *Guḍa-Mara* (jaggery killer), bot. name : *Gymnema sylvestrae*, as well as *Bilva* (*Aegle marmelos*). Pure honey does not harm patients with diabetes :

A special medicine in serious cases of diabetes is *Vasanta Kusumākara*. *Vasanta Kusumākara* is made as follows :

2 parts gold (revitalises)
2 parts silver (nerves)
3 parts tin
3 parts lead
3 parts iron
4 parts mercury
4 parts mica
4 parts coral
4 parts pearl

Triturate for seven days in one after the other of the following :

Cow's milk
Sugarcane juice
Vāsa (*Adhatoda vasica*)
Lotus (flower)
Turmeric
Rose
Jasmin
Camphor
Banana (rhizome)
Musk
+7 more substances.

This is the best for curing chronic diabetes. It is given for 6 months. It will take a month to start working on blood sugar. The medicine has a very heating effect.

7. MEDO ROGA (Adiposity)

Causes

Lack of exercise, sleep during day, intake of food aggravating K regularly, much sweet and fattening food, hereditary tendencies.

Pathogenesis

Because of taking much food with no exercise, the enzymes located in the channels carrying *Medas* stop functioning. So there is more of *Medas* accumulation, instead of the *Medas* going to *Asthi*, *Majjā* and *Śukra*.

There is much thirst, weakness and sweating and bad body odour, lack of strength and ability to work. Fat accumulates in the buttocks, the abdomen, the breasts etc.

Excess of adiposity can give rise to other diseases : fistula, piles, diabetes, liver disorders, skin problems, elephantiasis, for instance.

Treatment

Give less of fat, sugar, no yoghurt (because it obstructs circulation). Enzymes in channels must be stimulated.

Give barley and buckwheat and also wheat, but no rice, molasses instead of sugar.

Honey may be given in hot water. (This is the only case where this is permitted, since this reduces fat, otherwise honey is never given in hot drinks, this would have an extremely drying effect).

All pungent and bitter things are good, particularly the "three pungent drugs" (*trikaṭu*) very useful is also *Triphalā*.

All effective recipes revolve around : *Trikaṭu*
Triphalā
Honey.

Trimada is a standard medicine for reducing adiposity, this consists of :

Mustā (*Cyperus rotundus*)
Citraka (*Plumbago zeylanica*)
Viḍaṅga (*Embelia ribes*).

Guggulu reduces adiposity, a very popular remedy is : *Navaka Guggulu*, which consists of nine drugs in three groups of three each :

1. *Trimada* : *Mustā*, *Citraka*, *Viḍaṇga*.
2. *Triphalā* : *Harītakī*, *Bihītakī*, *Āmalakī*.
3. *Trikaṭu* : *Śuṇṭhī*, *Marica*, *Pippalī*.
4. *Guggulu* (*purified*).

Also useful are : Iron in *bhasma* form. Iron is very ununctuous, it is soaked in several drugs which are unuctuous.
Śilājatu.
Honey.

The patient should do strenuous exercises and be kept busy. He should not sleep during the day and stay up late night. Rice and white flour should be removed from the diet.

8. ARŚAS (Piles or Haemorrhoids)

This disesase is called : "The disease which gives you trouble like a constant enemy."

It is of six types : 1) V,
2) P,
3) K,
4) *Sannipāta*,
5) *Sahaja* (Congenital or hereditary), this is difficult to cure,
6) *Rakta* (Bleeding piles).

At times the veins in the lower rectal or anal will get varicosed and this gives rise to piles. Nasal polyps are a similar manifestation. All polyps, including warts, are included under *arśas*.

External haemorrhoids are easy to cure, internal ones difficult to cure.

Site of origin : Colon. Chyle from there goes to liver and heart.

Site of manifestation : rectum and anus.

V plays an important role in the pathogenesis of this disease.

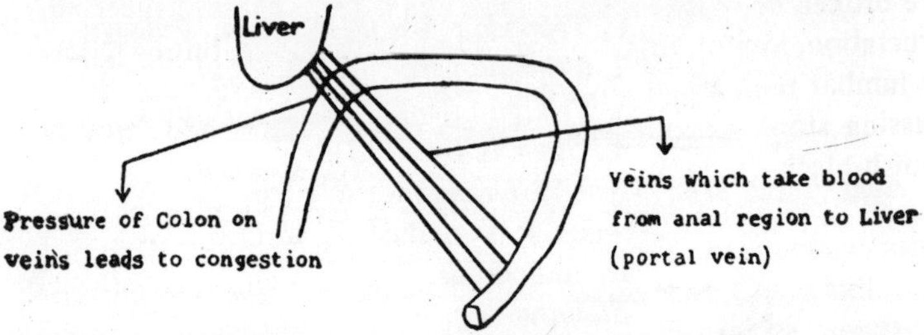

The veins get congested and the first swellings appear, tubular vessels take a round shape, fat, skin and tissue around the anus are involved with V.

Causes

V type : Excess of pungent, bitter and astringent things as food, ununctuous food,
cold food,
food with sharp qualities, alcohol in excess,
sex indulgence in excess immediately after food,
excessive fasting,
mental worry.

P type : Excess of pungent, sour and hot things as food,
excessive exposure to hot sun or fire,
anger,
heavy, indigestible food, hot drinks.

K type : Excess of sweet, unctuous and heavy food,
lack of exercise,
sleep during the day,
irresponsible life.

Sānnipātika type : If all the three mentioned above come together.

Rakta (bleeding) type : Same causes as P type.

Premonitory signs

Wind, lethargy, distension in lower abdomen, emaciation, eructation, less amount of stool, suspicion to get diarrhoea or intestinal disorder, loss of appetite, itching of the anus and often lumbago.

The different types

V type : there is a rough pile mass of different types, some are broken or cracked, some look like dates. There is sneezing, eructation, loss of appetite, loss of digestive power, tinnitus, pain in lumbar region and abdomen. Much sound and pain while passing stool, constipation, black stool. Skin will become bluish-black in colour, finger nails are blue, eyes bluish.

P *type* : the pile mass is slightly blue, red or yellow, and the piles exudate, they are not dry like in the V typc. The piles look like pieces of liver and will be hanging. There is burning sensation, fever, sweating, thirst, laziness. The stool is liquid and eiher black, yellow or red, hot to touch. The eyes are yellow, the urine is more yellow than usual.

K *type* : piles are hard to the touch and greasy, round in shape, heavy and immobile, there is slimy material. Feeling of cold in the pile mass. There is itching, pain in the lower pelvis and loss of appetite, salivation. Stool as if mixed with mucus or phlegm, anaemia will set in.

Hereditary piles may be V, P, K, or S. The K type is easier to cure, the S type the most difficult to cure, rather incurable.

Apāna-Vāyu is affected in case of piles.

Treatment

Very useful are: Jaggery (but not sugar)
Guggulu
Sesame seeds
Harītakī
Ginger (only in K type)
Amorphollus campanulatus (*sūraṇa*), rhizome
Benincasa hispida (a white pumpkin from which Agra *Peṭhā* is made). The pulp of this is good for bleeding, especially bleeding piles.

Make a paste of jaggery and sesame seeds, then add a

little *Harītakī*. You may follow this by milk. A little ginger may also be added to the jaggery and sesame seeds.

Abhayāriṣṭa, an alcoholic drink made with *Harītakī*, jaggery and some fragrant drugs is very useful for all six types. One ounce is given twice daily after food with an equal quantity of water.

Kāśīsādi taila, of which *kāśīsa* or iron sulphate is the important ingredient is used externally. This shrinks the piles and cures the itching. It relieves pain and checks bleeding.

Diet and Regimens

Curd with salt and cummin seed powder is useful.

Buttermilk with cummin seed and rock salt.

All foods which are good for liver and bowels. No fried food which would upset liver. Reduce consumption of alcohol.

Drākṣāsava, an alcoholic drink made from dry grapes is useful. Add seeds of *Plantago ovata* to this.

Goat milk and goat meat, vinegar and buttermilk are recommended.

For K type: Ginger and black pepper.

External : fumigation with human hair and snake skin, apply sesame oil with iron sulphate.

No excessive sex.

No horse riding.

No hard seats.

Frequent fasting is bad for piles, fasting always aggravates V, and there will be no refuse.

A note about yoghurat and frozen foods : frozen foods have less of *agni-mahābhūta*, these foods have a tendency to obstruct circulation channels.

Yoghurt obstructs channels of circulation. Yoghurt is good for *Sanyāsis* who live celebate, since it depresses sex, while milk stimulates sex.

Sour things are cardiac tonics.

If yoghurt is mixed 1 : 4 with water it is free from butter.

9. DIṚṢṬIDOṢA (Eyesight Disturbances, Refraction Errors)

Causes

1. Constipation, particularly in children can lead to bad eyesight.
2. Common cold, Rhinitis, Sinusitis.
3. General weakness.
4. Improper posture and bad light during studies.

Curative drugs should therefore be strength promoting, rejuvenating and against cold and constipation.

Treatment

Triphalā is very effective. The powder is soaked in water in a tumbler, the next morning the mixture is strained and honey is added. This is very good for children. First there may be a few untimely motions, constipation is cured. Cold and sinusitis are influenced favourably, weakness is removed and eyesight improves.

If there is cataract development, take this mixture for 2-3 months, this will improve the condition.

Triphalā Ghṛta : *Triphalā* boiled in cow's ghee, a medicated ghee, to which a few natural flavours are added. It is taken in a cup of warm cow's milk.

Saptāmṛta Lauha is very useful in cases of progressive myopia.

The name means "Sevenfold Nectar", since it consists of seven ingredients :

1-3 *Triphalā*.

4. *Yaṣṭīmadhu* (liquorice, which is always good for eyesight and joints).
5. Iron in *bhasma* form.
6. Honey.
7. Cow's ghee.

Mix equal quantities of 1-5, and then give 1 teaspoon mixed with honey and ghee. This is also good for chronic cold, sinusitis etc.

For retinal haemorrhage : coral in *bhasma* form is used for 2-3 months. This stops bleeding.

Rose water (cooling effect) + a little camphor added corrects many eye troubles.

Antimony as a collirium with ghee is good for eyes. As a substitute soot of a castor oil lamp can be used.

Very good honey applied to the conjunctiva is good. Put only 1 drop once a day. The honey collected from lotus blossoms is particularly good.

10. ŚIRAḤ ŚŪLA (Headache).

Headache is of 8 types :
1) V (instability in gait)
2) P (burning sensation)
3) K (with cough, cold, sinusitis)
4) *Sānnipātika*
5) *Ananta Vāta* (Migraine), involving pain all over the head usually coupled with nausea, giddiness.
6) *Śaṁkhaka* (Pain confined to temporal region, which swell and become red)
7) *Ardhāvabhedaka* (pain in half of the head)
8) *Sūryāvarta* (headache following the sunpath)

Causes

Physical as well as psychic factors are considered to be responsible for this disease. Responsible may be: defective eyesight, inflammation of the sinus, high blood pressure, sleeplessness, brain tumors, overwork, emotional strain, exposure of head to excessive heat cold or sun radiation, indigestion, constipation and wind formation, inflammatory stages, abrupt climatic changes; headache may be a symptom of fever, influenza, bronchitis etc. Signs and symptoms depend on the domination of the *doṣas* involved.

Signs and Symptoms

V type : giddiness, sleeplessness, dryness and roughness of eyes and various types of pain in different organs of the head.

P type : always associated with burning pain, inflammations, sometimes bleeding from nose.

K type : heaviness of head, watering of eyes, inflammation of middle ear, running nose, inflammation of mucous membrane of nose, nasal polyps etc.

Ananta Vāta: pain starts from the back of the head and migrated to the frontal as well as temporal regions.

Sūryāvarta: the headache starts in the morning and goes on increasing as the sun rises till midday, after which it decreases as the sun comes down again.

Treatment

Since the origin often lies in the colon, the bowels should be clean, give a purgative.

Medicated enemas are useful. Make these with almond oil and keep for half an hour.

If the enema gets absorbed in the meantime, this is good, since V will not find a place due to its greasiness. If there is much constipation, use castor oil.

If P is aggravated : add butter or ghee to the enema.

If K is aggravated: add ginger powder or honey.

If all 3 *doṣas* are aggravated: give a *Triphalā* enema.

In *Ananta Vāta* (migraine) usually P is involved. Heat almond oil, eventually boil it for a short period to take out the water, put into nose when slightly warm.

A medicine similar to the action of aspirin: Calcium Sulphate (Feldspar) given in *bhasma* form. (1g 2-3 times per day).

If K dominant: *Lakṣhmīvilāsa* (Mercury, Sulphur, Aconite etc.), taken internally with honey.

If P dominant: *Sūtaśekhara* (this is with *Āmalakī*).

If V dominant: *Lakṣhmīvilāsa* + Mica in *bhasma* form. The mica is roasted 100 times, it is given with a little ghee, milk or butter.

In *Sānnipātika* type: Gold preparations are given (gold in *bhasma* form).

Preparations containing gold often have the adjective

"*mahā*" before the name. *Mahā* means "great", so for instance *Mahā Lakṣhmī Vilāsa*.

If P is very dominant: *Svarna Sūtaśekhara* (Gold-*Sūtaśekhara*) which also corrects the stomach and gastric ulcers.

If V is very dominant: *Bṛhat Vāta Cintāmaṇī*, which corrects V.

Diet

This should be light, non-constipative. No yoghurt, no cold food, much honey.

Meditation and *yoga* exercises are very useful in many kinds of headaches.

11. AŚMARI (Stone in Urinary Tract)

Urinary stones are formed by calcium, phosphates or oxalates. Stones are formed primarily in the kidneys and may remain there unnoticed for a long time. Under certain circumstances they are dislodged and dissolved, because of this process they get lodged in a narrow part of the tract and cause excruciating pain.

Causative factors

Stones are formed because of V, which creates dryness in the body because of which the chemicals accumulate over a nucleus. This ultimately takes the shape of a stone. In this way at times the entire kidney can become calcified.

There are four types of stones: V, P, K, and *śukra* type.

K is always involved in *sāmānya samprāpti* (general pathogenesis), K is visciated and gets dried up by V. So V and K are there in the pathogenesis of the disease, V taking its origin from the colon.

Origin

The disease takes its origin in the colon, then circulates through the channels of *Rasa* and gets located in the kidney, bladder, uretera etc. The kidney is enlarged, finally stops functioning and there is more urea, more uric acid enters the blood.

To compensate, the other kidney also enlarges, it is not uncommon to have stones in both the kidneys.

Śukra type: prostratic secretion goes to the bladder (it does not contain sperm)

Signs and Symptoms

Pain in the lumber, navel and pelvic region, urination problems, different colours of urine, bleeding with urine. The pain radiates towards the genital organs. There might be fever vomiting, loss of appetite, sleeplessness and painful urination.

V type : Tremendous pain, agony. Urine comes in drops, pale yellow urine.

P type: Urine is very hot, burning sensation in pelvic region, stone will be black in colour.

K type: Urine in large quantity, milky in colour, specific gravity will be higher.

Śukra type: Urine will contain a lot of sediments. (Retention of semen inside body). Terrible pain in pelvic region, swelling of testicles, passing *Śarkarā* (graveluria), extreme fatigue, anorexia, emaciated and anaemic condition, patient is very thirsty, pain in cardiac region. (Heart and kidneys are interconnected). Heart, kidneys and brain are vital organs (*Marma-traya*).

Treatment

The first step is to take care of the constipation. But if patient is weak, so we cannot give strong purgatives. If *Apāna Vāyu* is not affected, there will be no pain.

Give a medicated enema of castor oil, this is soothing and evacuating, although it is only a temporary measure.

The next step is either to dissolve the stone or to remove it by operation.

(Āyurvedic surgery of stone in the bladder is described).

Drugs for Dissolving

1. *Pāṣāṇa Bheda* (*Bergenia ligulata* or *Bergenia ciliata*). Rhizome as powder or decoction.
2. *Gokṣura* (*Tribulus terrestris*), decoction of tea, twice daily Diuretic.

3. *Śilājatu* (asphalt). Strong therapautic for urino-genital tract.
4. *Varuṇa* (*Cretiva religiosa*)
5. *Guggulu* (*Commiphora mukul*). Helps in alleviation of *Vāyu*.
6. *Badara Pāṣāṇa*.

Cystone is a patent medicine containing all the six ingredients mentioned above.

Kulattha-(*Dolichos biflorus*), is a dal suitable for making soups. After the stone is out, give this *dal*.

Diet and Regimens

Take barley, barley water, meat from arid zones, white pumpkin as vegetable, ginger.

Don't take any constipating or wind forming food, avoid beans and pulses.

Spinach at times causes wind formation but in some individuals it also acts as a laxative.

Cauliflower also causes wind formation, therefore add garlic and ginger to it.

Tomatoes are bad in case of oxalate stones.

Tender radish causes wind, also potatoes.

Take fruit juice in good quantity.

To reduce wind: give Asafoetida, garlic and ginger, also *Aloe vera* juice.

The patient should not sit continuously for a long time. Immediately after taking food he should either walk or lie down for a few minutes. After working about an hour the patient should move about for a few minutes. Avoid constipation, therefore a laxative should be taken practically every day. Plenty of water should be drunk to help him to micturate frequently. This will cleanse the urinary system.

Stones will break down into small fragments and come out, if the patient is treated correctly.

12. RAKTA CĀPA VṚDDHI (High Blood Pressure)

Causes: V dries up the elasticity of the blood vessels, due to constant intake of food which aggravates V, as well as mental stress and worry. Constipation, suppression of urine and faeces, vitiate *Apāna Vāyu*. Heart and blood channels get affected. (Remember the Heart-kidney relation). High blood pressure can also start right from the heart. In case of much worry the liver and kidneys are affected.

Origin: this disease also originates in the colon, so take care of this. Mental conditions count very much, stress has to be reduced.

Treatment

Hypotensive drugs may produce toxicity and only temporary relief.

Instead give a medicated enema with castor oil, sesame oil, 4 ounces every third day.

Triphalā powder is to be taken regularly. (1 teaspoon in a tumbler of water, next morning strain and drink. *Āma* in the blood gets dislodged in this way and comes back through motion. Continue this treatment for 3 months at least.

Take care of good sleep. There is sleeplessness due to V, simultaneously sleeplessness causes V. V sleeplessness, is a vicious circle.

Brāhmī will bring sleep in many cases. Massage the soles of the feet, add an equal quantity of water, massage also the head.

The root of long pepper brings sleep.

Another recipe: take a ripe banana, cut the centre and add cummin seeds and take at bed time.

Drugs recommended

1. *Brāhmī*, will bring sleep in many cases. Add equal quantity of water and massage soles and head.
2. *Vacā* (*Acorus calamus*).
3. *Jaṭāmāṁsī* (*Nardostachys jatamansī*).
4. *Valeriana wallichu*.

5. *Sarpagandhā* (*Rauwolfia serpentina*) the root. Add this to the other drugs.

A readily obtainable medicine is Santab, which contains the medicines mentioned above except *Sarpagandhā*. A stronger variety called Santab (Forte) which however contains *Sarpagandhā* as well.

Sarpagandhā was discovered through the study of Ayurvedic texts by the German physician Rauwolf, during the 16th century. The species which is named after him : *Rauwolfia Serpentina*, known as snake root, became the point of departure of a number of Western drugs used to lower blood pressure. (Reserpine, the alkaloid which the species contains, is a strong antihypertensive and sedative). While Western medicine isolated this alkaloid, Āyurvedic medicine continued to administrate *Sarpagandhā* as a whole. The destruction of the highly complex totality of the phytocomplex of a species through analytical separation is alien to Āyurveda.

13. VICARCIKĀ (Eczema)

Eczema is an acute or chronic, noncontagious, itching, inflammatory disease of the skin; the skin is reddened, the redness shading off into the surrounding unaffected parts. According to Western medicine the cause is unknown. Eruptions of similar appearance due to ingested drugs or local irritants are referred to as dermatitis medicamentosa, contact dermatitis or dermatitis venenata. (From Blackiston's Medical Dictionary)

Causative Factors

Food and drinks which are contradictory.

Excessively heavy food.

Suppression of natural urges, particularly vomiting.

Exercise immediately after food.

Changing from hot to cold or from cold to hot environment rapidly.

Eating freshly harvested corn, sour things and fish in excess.

Sex before food is digested.

Not showing respect for people who are worthy of respect

Improper metabolism.

Affected lymphatics.

Not undergoing the five eliminations (*Pañca Karma*) when necessary.

In *Sāmānya Samprāpti* all three *doṣas* are involved.

Skin, muscle tissue, lymphatics and eventual presence of germs must be corrected.

Line of Treatment

Correct food habits and sinful acts, clean the system of waste products. Many skin diseases are psychosomatic, therefore the body and the mind must be treated.

The waste products must be taken out from the body, therefore the bowels have to be cleaned.

1. Strong purgatives are given to the patient.
2. Correct the blood and lymphatics. The controlling organ of the lymphatics is the liver. So give medicines which correct the function of the liver. i.e. bitter drugs. Bitter substances will remove impurities from the blood and correct the functioning of the liver.

   Avoid yoghurt, since it will obstruct the channels of circulation.

   Don't take salt in case of skin diseases, if salt has to be given then give rock salt.

Medicines to be given

These are of two kinds : 1. External, to kill germs and to heal skin lesions.

2. Internal, (bitter drugs) for blood purification, purgation and for correcting liver function.

Khadira (*Acacia catechu*).

Nimba (*Margosa indica*).

There are many preparations containing these two drugs.

Haridrā (turmeric).

Aloe vera are also very effective if applied externally.

Sulphur, which is purified in the Āyurvedic sense, is made into an ointment with vaseline or bee's wax. This kills germs.

The prepared sulphur is also used internally for correcting the liver, the *doṣas,* against waste products and for the purification of the blood.

(Take 100 mg twice daily with honey in empty stomach. Ready made Āyurvedic medicines of this type are also available).

Sulphur is of hot potency, therefore do not expose the patient to much sun. If too much of S or Hg enters the blood, this may cause a rash.

To correct this rash, the pulp of coconut is best. The rash effect due to S or Hg is rare however, but it may appear.

S is normally good for K *Prakṛti* people. But an adverse effect is found in P *Prakṛti* people only.

Emetic therapy is given in empty stomach, not after eating. After this give :

1st day : thin gruel.

2nd day : thick gruel.

3rd and 4th days : vegetable soup.

5th and 6th days : meat soup.

7th day : food.

The first meal after vomiting must always be light.

Gandhaka Rasāyana : a tonic prepared from Sulphur. Give 1 teaspoon twice daily with hot milk or honey.

If the eczema is not cured : an

Arsenic preparation is given. There is white arsenic, yellow arsenic (orpiment) and red arsenic (realgar).

To prepare yellow arsenic : soak yellow arsenic in the juice of white pumpkin for seven days. (This white pumpkin juice is also given in case of arsenic poisoning). After soaking, the arsenic is triturated, dried, and the process repeated. This is done 7 times. The powder of this purified arsenic is kept inside two mica sheets and then heated on an oven.

Fumes will appear, these should not be inhaled since they are harmful. The mica is turned over by a spatula, more smoke will come out. When the smoke ceases, let it cool down. A beautiful red layer called

Rasa Māṇikya will be formed. Mix 100 mg with honey and ghee together and take.

Don't give this medicine to people in summer.

Honey and milk should be given in large quantities, and also ghee. Preferably no salt, if salt is given, then only rock-salt.

Caṇḍa Mārutham is a Siddha medicine. This is a preparation of mercury and arsenic. (The name of this medicine actually means Hanuman in a state of terrible anger.) Don't give this medicine in summer. The patient may need 2-3 courses of treatment with this medicine. There are side effects: salivation, ulcers in the urethra and the mouth, difficulty in passing stool, ulcers in all mucous joints and eyelids. For correcting the side effects use the pulp of coconut, just like in the case of Sulphur.

Soap is bad in cases of eczema and other skin diseases. Instead use chick pea flour to clean the body.

14. HṚDROGA (Heart Disease)

The heart is the seat of the mind and the source of life (*Prāṇa vāyu*). The heart is one of the 3 vital organs (heart, kidneys, brain).

There are five kinds of heart diseases :

1. V
2. P
3. K
4. S
5. *Kṛmija* (caused by infection).

Heart diseases are most serious forms of disorder and much knowledge is needed for treating them successfully. For the time being we shall only discuss some supporting medicines :

1. *Arjuna* (*Terminalia arjuna*). This is a big tree, from the bark tea or alcoholic drink (*ariṣṭa*) is made. *Ariṣṭas* are always taken after food.

2. Mica (*Abhraka*) is the best mineral for the heart (in *bhasma* form).
3. Gold. This is cold in potency, although it is dominated by *agni mahābhūta*.

   Sevaral preparations with mica and gold are used for heart diseases, common is *Yogendra Rasa*, which is also used for nervous disorders. Give one pill twice daily with honey.
4. Pearl tones up the heart muscle, it is also good to wear pearls externally.

Nāgārjunābhraka is a preparation containing mica and *arjuna*. Give 1 pill in the morning and one in the evening.

The mentioned medicines are not effective in case of congenital defects, for instance a foramen will not be closed.

V is predominant in heart diseases (*prāṇa* and *udāna*), don't aggravate V by food etc.

Avoid too much stress, regulate the diet, take care of wind formation.

Only mild purgatives are given. Wind should have a downward movement.

15. ŚŪLA (Colic pain)

Colic pain can be caused by several factors : gastritis, ulcers, appendicitis, stones in the kidneys or gall bladder, intestinal spasms etc.

We treat the painful symptoms, after this there is urgent need for investigation.

Correct the V of pain. (Oil, ghee, purgatives, enema, the last two both with oils.)

Gently massage the abdomen of the patient.

Conch Shell *Bhasma* or a Cowrie Shell preparation are useful. (The small yellowish Cowries which are heavy are the best).

Method of preparation of Cowrie Shell medicine :

Put one Cowrie Shell in a bottle of lemon juice (about 4

ounces of juice), the Cowrie dissolves, add a little rock-salt. Give half a teaspoon of this mixture to the patient. The preparation remains active for 6 months.

A method of preparation of Conch Shell *bhasma* : This shell is triturated in vinegar, then heated over fire. After this again triturate in vinegar and proceed as before. This process is repeated 7 times. The result should not be caustic, if it is caustic triturate in milk.

Give 1 g of this powder mixed with honey or water, 2-3 times per day.

If there is pain all over, the condition is V.

If there is burning sensation and emaciation, the condition is P.

If there is vomiting and nausea, the condition is K.

In case of V and P : Cowrie is more effective.

In case of K : Conch is more effective.

Sometimes the two powders are mixed. Conch and Cowrie are both hot in potency, they show immediate action.

In case of P condition, add coral or pearl powder to the Cowrie. Pearl, coral, mother of pearl are cooling.

Coral and pearl are rubbed with rose water for about 1 month. *Bhasma* reduces the cooling effect.

The seeds of plantago (all varieties) can be given in hot milk at bedtime. The husk of these is specially effective. This is also good in diarrhoea, except that it is to be given in buttermilk or yoghurt instead of milk. The seeds should be crushed for greater effectiveness.

16. PRATIŚYĀYA (Common cold)

"The common cold is a mild, acute, contagious upper respiratory viral infection of short duration, characterized by coryza (inflammation of the mucous membranes of the nose)[1] watering of the eyes, cough and occasionally, fever."

(Blakiston's Pocket Medical Dictionary, p. 185).

---

1. Inflammation of the mucous membranes of the nose is also called Rhinitis.

Precipitating Causes

Exposure to cold, cold drinks, abrupt changes of environmental temperature etc.

Pratiśyāya is of 4 types : V, K, P and S.

1. V type : there is pain all over, specially strong in the head.
2. K type: there is much sneezing, mucus watering of the eyes and heaviness of head.
3. P type : the nose is blocked, burning sensation of nose, dry sneezing.
4. S type : this is more serious, there is fever and cough as well.

Site of origin : stomach.

If a cold is neglected it may turn into sinusitis (inflammation of a sinus).

If further neglected, it may turn into chronic cough or asthma specially bronchial asthma.

Treatment

Fasting, light diet, no sleep during daytime.

Ginger, black pepper long pepper in equal quantity together to make 1/4 spoon.

To this *Trikaṭu* a little honey may be added, this corrects the stomach, which is the site of origin of the trouble.

Inhaling of eucalyptus vapour is excellent.

If the cold is of more chronic nature, instil 2 drops of mustard oil into the nose, this is a little irritating.

Turmeric powder can be taken 2 or 3 times (a teaspoon) mixed with hot milk.

It is not useful to give a purgative since a purgative is only effective when the body can release *āma*. Therefore no purgative is given in the beginning.

After a few days purgatives can be given.

Add *trikaṭu* to soups as well.

Later give anything alleviating K, purgation or even better emesis will be useful. Give 5-6 glasses of saltwater, the *yogic kriya* of kunjal is useful.

Ready Medicines

Lakṣmīvilāsa : a combination of mercury, sulphur, black pepper aconite and borax. Stronger than this is :

Nāradīya Lakṣmīvilāsa, in which in places of aconite *dhatūra* (*kanaka*) is added, this has a very drying effect. If after a long time conditions have become chronic, and chronic sinusitis etc. have set in : give—

Mahālakṣmīvilāsa which is *Lakṣmīvilāsa*+gold, which makes the effect more potent.

Amṛta Dhārā is a useful recipe of camphor, menthol and thymol.

Cyavanaprāśa is also very useful.

Harītakī does not work in acute stages of cold.

17. Notes on Massage

Svedana and *Snehana* (Fomentation and Oleation) should always be given to a patient before *Pañca karma* treatment. Thus the order of *Pañca karma* is :

Preparation :
1. *Snehana* (Oleation including massage).
2. *Svedana* (Fomentation).

Pañca karma:
1. *Vamana* (Emesis).
2. *Virecana* (Purgation).
3. *Nirūha* (medicated enema with decoctions of drugs).
4. *Anuvāsana* (unctuous enema preparation with oils or other unctuous substances).
5. *Nasya* (Inhalation therapy).

Unctuous substances are :
1. different oils (*taila*), ghee (*ghṛta*).
2. fat collected from animals (*vasā*).
3. Fat from bone marrow (*majjā*).

Taila, oil is the least greasy.
ghṛta, ghee, is more greasy.
vasā, animal fat is still more greasy and
majjā, bone marrow, is the most greasy.

All these have their own particular properties.

If drugs are boiled in *taila* or *ghṛta*, the preparation will carry medical properties of the drugs used.

For massage generally oil is used, this is cheap and effective for V conditions. In very cold countries (for instance Mongolia) animal fats are used.

Massage with sesame oil alleviates V, almond oil tones up the nervous system.

Some standard rules on massage oils

1. For fatigued persons who desire more strength : *Nārāyaṇa Taila*, an oil containing many herbs.
2. For patients with much pain all over the body, pain in general, V minus *Āma* : Use *Nārāyaṇa Taila* as well, or *Mahānārāyaṇa Taila*, which is stronger but a little more greasy.
3. For patients with pain in the joints (rheumatism), i.e. V plus *Āma* : Use *Saindhavādi Taila*.
4. In case of burning sensation, sleeplessness, P aggravated: *Bhṛṅgarāja* (*Eclipta alba*) or *Brāhmī Taila*.

   A simple massage in case of sleeplessness; use sesame oil and water, massage hands and feet soles. But *Bhṛṅgarāja* is very effective.
5. For patients with skin trouble: *Kuṣṭharākṣasa Taila*.

Almond oil is used in all cases where toning up of the nervous system is desired, (emotional problems, drugs etc.)

Massage can be given every day if there is much pain.

It is given from the centre to the periphery, from the heart outwards, and from up to down, not down to up as in some modern system of physio-therapy.

If massage is given, away from the heart, metabolic waste in the blood will come out through sweat.

Massage produces heat. No bath or air exposure immediately afterwards is allowed. After half an hour's rest, a hot water bath or shower can be taken. The head is bathed only, with luke warm water. Hot water would be harmful in this case.

To a hot bath for *svedana*, castor leaves should be added to the hot water.

Excessive oil after massage should be removed not with soap but with chick pea flour (*besaun*).

Pīlī Miṭṭī (an Indian yellow clay) is excellent for washing, it has a cooling effect and soothes the nerves.

18. Notes on Some Excellent Drugs and Regimens

1. WATER is the best for producing soothing effect.
2. WINE is the best to dispel fatigue.
3. MILK is the best to invigorate.
4. MEAT is the best nourishing, but not necessary for people who are already nourished. Be careful with overnourishment.
5. MEAT SOUP is the best for refreshing.
6. SALT is the best to cause deliciousness of food.
7. COCK'S MEAT is the best to promote strength. (not chicken).
8. HONEY is the best to alleviate *Kapha*.
9. BUTTER " *Pitta*
10. SESAME OIL " *Vāyu*
11. EMESIS " *Kapha*
12. PURGATION " *Pitta*
13. ENEMA " *Vāyu*
14. FOMENTATION (13 types) is the best to cause tenderness. (Sauna bath, warm salt over body etc.)
15. EXERCISE, including YOGIC EXERCISE, is the best to bring sturdiness of the body. Yogic exercise also brings flexibility of the spine.
16. ALKALIES cause impotency. (They promote digestion however, but don't use too long).
17. GOAT MILK is the best for tuberculosis and bleeding.
18. CAMEL MILK is the best for curing water accumulation in abdomen and cirrhosis of liver.
19. COW'S MILK is the healthiest milk, and butter made from it is the best butter. It is also excellent for cheese.
20. BUFFALO MILK is the best for producing sleep.

21. *MADANA* (*Randia dumetorum*) is the best for emesis (add a little powder to water).
22. *TRIVṚT* (*Operculina turpethum*) is the best as a painless prugative which purifies.
23. *ĀRAGVADHA* (*Cassia fistula*) is the best laxative. Take the pulp of the pod (seeds taken out). It is suitable even for pregnant women.
24. *APĀMĀRGA* (*Achryanthes aspera*) is the best for the elimination of phlegm from the head. The root is also inhaled in case of sinusitis.
25. *ŚIRIṢA* (*Albizia lebbeck*) is the best anti-toxic medicine. (Decoction of bark).
26. BARLEY is the best to increase faeces.
27. *KHADIRA* (*Acacia catechu*) is the best for blood. Take along with betel leaf. Also used in cases of diabetes.
28. *RĀSNĀ* (*Pluchea lanceolata*) is the best to alleviate *Vāyu*.
29. *ĀMALAKA* (*Emblica officinalis*) is the best rejuvenator.
30. *HARĪTAKĪ* is the best having wholesome effect.
31. *CITRAKA* (*Plumbago zeylanica*) is the best digestive (root).
32. *ERAṆḌA* (*Ricinus communis*) is the best to alleviate rheumatism.
33. *PUṢKARAMŪLA* (*Inula racemosa*) is the best for asthma.
34. *MUSTĀ* (*Cyperus rotundus*) is the best to stop diarrhoea (small nodules at roots).
35. *ATIVIṢĀ* (*Aconitum heterophyllum*) is the best for causing astringent effect.
36. *PRIYAṄGU* (*Callicarpa macrophylla*) is the best drug for stopping excessive menstrual bleeding.
37. *KUṬAJA* (*Hollarhena antidysenterica*) is the best for fever and chronic diarrhoea.
38. *GOKṢURA* (*Tribulus terrestris*) is the best for urinary disorders and burning micturition.
39. NUTMEG (*Myristica fragrans*) is good for teething babies. Give 125 mg twice daily. Remove hard shell and make a powder. Can be taken in milk or honey.
40. FRESH AIR is the best life giver.
41. TAKING FOOD IN TIME is the best healthy practice.
42. TRANQUILITY OF MIND is the best regimen.

43. CELIBACY is the best for long life.
44. UNHAPPINESS is the most important factor for losing virility.
45. GRIEF, the most important factor for aggravation of diseases.
46. CHEERFULNESS is the best nourishment for happiness.
47. WORRY is the most important emaciating factor.
48. OLD GHEE (kept for 5 years or more) is the best for insanity.
49. GINGER (*Zingiber officinale*) is best for chronic indigestion (with rock-salt), when taken 5 minutes before food. (Fresh ginger): Continue this for 2 months.

19. The Classical Regimens for Day and Night

Sukhārthāḥ sarva bhūtānām
Yataḥ sarve pravrttayaḥ
Sukham ca na vinā dharmāt
Tasmāt dharmaparo bhavet.

(All efforts of man's aim at getting happiness, one can never achieve that aim without *dharma*. Therefore, one should follow religious prescriptions.)

In accordance with this idea, life in India had and still has its set rules for the day and the night.

Getting up in the morning one should first remember God or a Saint.

Then wash your face with cold water, keeping water in the mouth during washing.

Then drink a glass of water on empty stomach.

Go to the toilet for ablutions.

Brush the teeth. Massage the gums well. This is good for eyesight. Use herbal power, sticks or tooth paste. Astringent taste is useful. Brush teeth morning and evening.

Scrape the tongue. This takes out dirt and is also good for eyesight. Scrapers are available in gold, silver, stainless steel, plastic and aluminium. Sesame oil boiled with *Acacia catechu*, put in warm water, is good for loose teeth. Also a tooth paste made from tobacco and jaggery settles loose teeth.

Coral powder and Conch Sheel *Bhasma* are good for teeth and bones.

20. How to make Śankha Bhasma (Conch Shell Bhasma) for teeth calcium

The Conch shell is cut and soaked in lemon juice. The conch must be free from impurities. Soak in the lemon juice for 7 days, then triturate. Make small round pills out of the paste. Keep these in an earthen plate or flat bowl, but another plate or bowl of the same kind over the lower one and smear the joint.

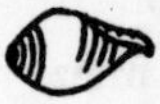

Fire this for 12 hours, cool overnight, next day fire another 4 hours, take the pills out the next day. Soak again for 1 day with lemon juice, again make pills, calcine as before (calcinatio occlusa). Do this at least 3 times, others insist that it has to be done 7 times.

For liver improvement : add *Aloe vera* juice (lemon juice is used only the first time in this case).

For constipation : add latex of *Calotropis gigantea* (laxative effect).

If the *bhasma* is caustic : soak in milk for 1 day.

Next go for massage, usually oil massage. This prevents aging and fatigue, and also makes the body sturdy. Sesame oil is good in summer, in winter a warmer oil is used for instance mustard oil. Cocount oil is not greasy.

Then take your bath or shower, avoid hot water on the head. The head should always be washed with cool water, this is good for sleep as well as eyesight.

Then dress correctly.

Use flowers and garlands, and perfume from different flowers.

Put on your ornaments, they are good for health, wear chains of gold, ear-rings etc.

Take your breakfast in a peaceful place, your attendants, guests and your animals must have their food first. The family or your wife or husband should be present. Do not discuss problems at breakfast.

Do not sleep during the day.

During the day avoid 10 shameful things:

1. Violence.
2. Desire for unnatural things.
3. Backbiting.
4. Harsh words.
5. Speaking lies.
6. Inconsistant speech and action.
7. Thinking ill of others.
8. Desire of the wealth of others.
9. Desire for other's wife or husband.
10. Don't deal improperly with friends and enemies.

During the night: take almonds, cow's milk and sugar after sex.

Index

183, 184

Fasting, 47, 73, 161, 163, 171, 182
Fat, 30, 33, 40, 132
Fatigue, 111
Fea, 40
Feces, 40
Ferula foetida Regel., 116
Ferula narthex Boiss., 116
Fever, 21, 46, 50, 56, 65, 97, 104, 112, 122, 124, 137, 142, 150, 169, 181, 184, 195
Fever, chronic, 107, 139
Fistula, 178
Flatulence, 116
Flatus, 45
Flour, white, 179
Foetus, 42
Fomentation, 45, 172, 197, 199
Foramen, 194
Fractures, 120, 177
Frozen foods, 182
Fumigation, 182
Fungicide, 102

Galactogogue, 109, 150
Gallbladder, 137
Gandhaka rasāyana, 192
Gāndharva prakṛti, 43
Gandha tanmātra, 12, 14
Garbha (embryo), 42
Garlands of flowers, 203
Garlic, 84, 102, 171, 187, 189
Gastritis, 194
Gastrointestinal tract, 109
Genus, 79
Genital organs, 13, 38, 45
Germs, 58, 59, 160, 192
Ghee, 73, 159, 162, 169, 183, 18?, 188, 193, 194, 197
Ghee, medicated, 78, 173
Ghee, old, 201
Ghrānendriya, 13
Ghṛta (ghee), 197
medicated, 78
Ginger, 73, 92, 97, 160, 161, 167, 169, 170, 172, 182, 185, 187, 188, 195, 201
Glaze of eyes, 33
Glycyrrhiza glabra, 76, 110
Goitre, 38, 120
Gokṣura (Tribulus terrestris), 151, 153, 177, 187, 200
Gold, 79, 163, 168, 177, 186, 194, 196
Gold śilājatu, 177
Gout, 147, 170
Gṛahaṇī (sprue syndrome), 50
Granuloma, 38
Grief, 40, 160, 201
Guḍa mara (Jaggery killer), 177
Guḍūcī (Tinospora cordifolia), 139
Guggulu (Commiphora molmol), 118, 171, 177, 179, 180, 188
Guṇas, 14, 42
Guru (heavy), 19, 26
Guṭika (pills), 78
Gymnema sylvestrae, 177

Haemoglobin, 30, 33
Haemopoetic, 101
Haemorrhage, 90
Haemorrhage, retinal, 183
Haemorrhoids, 124
external, 179
internal, 179
Hair, 27, 33, 87, 102, 138
Hair-follicles, 40
Hair, human, 182
Hand, 13
Hanuman, 193
Haridrā (turmeric), 97, 191
Haridrā-meha (turmeric meha), 176
Harītakī, 82, 84, 98, 166, 169, 170, 179, 181, 197, 200
Herītra, 7
Hasti-meha (elephant meha), 175
Headache, 45, 139, 184
sannipatika type of, 185
treatment of, 184
as a symptom, 184
Heart, 21, 22, 23, 37, 166, 169, 179, 189
Heart, disease, 69, 90, 94, 102, 104, 106, 115, 153, 193, 194
Heart, malfunctioning of, 46
Heart pain, 118
Heat, excessive, 185
exposure to, 40
Hemicrania, 46
Hereditary diseases, 48
Herpestris Monnieri, 103
Hiccup, 20, 46, 157, 158, 166
Hiñgu (ferula foetida Boiss, and Ferula narthex Regel.), 116, 166
Hingvaṣṭaka cūrṇa, 169
Hip-bone, 39, 170
Hippocrates, 2
Hollarhena antidysenterica, 200
Homocopathic medicine, 67, 130
Honey, 67, 73, 158, 161, 162, 166, 167, 177, 178, 179, 183, 186, 192, 194, 195, 197, 199
Hookworm, 137
Hormones, 120
Horripilation, 40
Hṛdroga (heart disease), 193
Hunger, 47
Hydrochloric acid, 32
Hydrocotyle asiatica, 103
Hyper cholesterolemia, 120
Hypotensive drugs, 189
Hysteria, 118

Iatro chemistry, 9
Ikṣu-meha (sugarcane meha), 174
Immunity, 188
Impotency, 37, 39
Incompatible food, 39